FACIAL DIAGNOSIS OF CELL SALT DEFICIENCY

FACIAL DIAGNOSIS
OF CELL SALT
DEFICIENCY

A User's Guide

DAVID R. CARD

Kalindi Press
Chino Valley, Arizona

Cover design: Kim Johansen
Layout and design: Tori Bushert

Kalindi Press
PO Box 4410
Chino Valley, AZ 86323
800-381-2700
www.kalindipress.com

This book was printed in China on recycled paper using soy ink.

Disclaimer: The material in this book is intended for educational purposes only, and as such is not meant to be a substitute for professional medical intervention or used to treat or diagnose diseases. In any use of cell salts or other approaches discussed in this book, please apply common sense and consult a qualified, licensed health care professional.

Dedication

This book is dedicated to the patience of my family, my clients, and my mentor, Dr. Robin Murphy.

Many thanks to Monique Ordonez for the cell salt allegory illustration, and to Linda Fulton for her typing, photography, and organization.

Thanks go to the memory of Dr. George Carey. His work has been simplified, reformatted, and adapted here for the twenty-first-century reader.

Contents

Introduction

Chapter 1   **Using Cell Salts — 1**
An introduction to cell salts, including dosages
and instructions for their use, and an overview
regarding facial deficiency diagnosis

Chapter 2   **Introduction and History — 10**
An introduction to and history of cell salt usage
by Dr. Carey; charts comparing cell salt attributes

Chapter 3   **CALC FLUOR — 17**
Introduction, *materia medica*, photographs and
descriptions of facial deficiencies, Schuessler's
recommended uses, astrological correspondences

Chapter 4   **CALC PHOS — 27**
Introduction, *materia medica*, photographs and
descriptions of facial deficiencies, Schuessler's
recommended uses, astrological correspondences

Chapter 5   **CALC SULPH — 39**
Introduction, *materia medica*, photographs and
descriptions of facial deficiencies, Schuessler's
recommended uses, astrological correspondences

Chapter 6   **FERRUM PHOS — 49**
Introduction, *materia medica*, photographs and
descriptions of facial deficiencies, Schuessler's
recommended uses, astrological correspondences

Chapter 7   **KALI MUR — 62**
Introduction, *materia medica*, photographs and
descriptions of facial deficiencies, Schuessler's
recommended uses, astrological correspondences

Chapter 8   **KALI PHOS — 74**
Introduction, *materia medica*, photographs
and descriptions of facial deficiencies, Schuessler's
recommended uses, astrological correspondences

Chapter 9   **KALI SULPH — 86**
Introduction, *materia medica*, photographs
and descriptions of facial deficiencies, Schuessler's
recommended uses, astrological correspondences

Chapter 10   **MAG PHOS — 96**
Introduction, *materia medica*, photographs
and descriptions of facial deficiencies, Schuessler's
recommended uses, astrological correspondences

Chapter 11   **NAT MUR — 107**
Introduction, *materia medica*, photographs
and descriptions of facial deficiencies, Schuessler's
recommended uses, astrological correspondences

Chapter 12   **NAT PHOS — 120**
Introduction, *materia medica*, photographs
and descriptions of facial deficiencies, Schuessler's
recommended uses, astrological correspondences

Chapter 13   **NAT SULPH — 130**
Introduction, *materia medica*, photographs
and descriptions of facial deficiencies, Schuessler's
recommended uses, astrological correspondences

Chapter 14   **SILICEA — 141**
Introduction, *materia medica*, photographs and
descriptions of facial deficiencies, Schuessler's
recommended uses, astrological correspondences

Appendix — 151

Glossary — 153

Bibliography — 157

Cell Salt Sources — 158

Index — 159

About the Author — 173

Introduction

Hopefully, through the photographs provided, this book will help you to visualize and recognize cell salt deficiencies and gain greater health.

There has been a great amount of interest in cell salts in the last few years. Most of the material in English is a rehash of the classics. I have updated two classic books from the 1920s written by Dr. George Carey. They are *The Biochemic System of Medicine* and *The Chemistry and Wonders of the Human Body*. I have adapted Dr. Carey's *materia medica* (a collection of symptom details) for the layperson, translating some of his older technical medical terms into more modern-day language. The Glossary at the end of the book will also assist you with terms that are unfamiliar.

Dr. Carey's reference material is immensely interesting and useful. In each chapter covering a particular cell salt, I provide this information as well as a *Reader's Digest*–type version of his other writings on that particular remedy. Included in Chapter 2 are also several pages of cell salt comparisons.

In Europe the use of cell salts and facial deficiency diagnosis is widespread. In Germany alone, there are about sixty "cell salt" organizations. The European view of cell salts originates from two followers of Dr. W. H. Schuessler – Dr. Kurt Hickethier and Mrs. W. Sonner, who established the Sonnerschau Facial Analysis Theory in 1936. Since that time, thousands of practitioners have verified their observation that facial features reflect the symptoms of cell salt deficiencies. In each chapter I provide material from Dr. Schuessler's "Therapeutic Index," which can be found in his book, *A New Treatment of Disease by the Inorganic Tissue Cell Salts*. I also include photographs and descriptions of cell salt deficiencies as seen in the face.

The last part of Dr. Carey's work has to do with his obsession with the cell salts and their relationship to the astrological constellations, birth times, and body parts. I include this information at the end of each chapter to provide a different view of the cell salts.

This book is not intended to treat or diagnose diseases. Please use common sense and consult your health care professional.

CHAPTER 1

Using Cell Salts

Cell salts can be taken by anyone under any condition. Because they are nontoxic, many pregnant and nursing women use them with success.

There are several ways to take cell salts. The most common way is to tap 2–4 pellets into the cap and drop them into the mouth. (Refer to page 2, "Use and Handling of Cell Salts.") This is called the "**dry**" **method**. Many people prefer this method, especially children who like sweet foods or candy.

Cell salts commonly have a lactose (milk sugar) base. Those with a lactose intolerance can purchase cell salts with a liquid or sucrose base, however they may be harder to obtain in these forms.

In chronic cases in which a person will be taking cell salts for several months or longer, you may have to alter the potency or use a "**wet**" **form**. This means that you put your pellets into a bottle of distilled or filtered water (8 to 64 ounces) and consume it throughout the day. The advantages of the wet form include the healing benefits of drinking pure water and continuously infusing the body with cell salts throughout the day.

There are different ideas regarding the amount of cell salts to be taken. Some people suggest 2–4 pellets taken 1–3 times a day. Acute cases seem to dictate 5–30 pellets 3 times a day. My approach is to use applied kinesiology to determine the potency and number of pellets one should take.

We have two types of mineral reserves in the body, one to use on a daily basis and one for emergency situations. When our local reservoirs are depleted, we must draw from our deeper wells. When we are deficient in minerals, this is reflected in the face as well as in diseases or imbalances. The greater the deficiency, the greater the changes in the face. (The photographs shown later in the book illustrate this principle.) When these signs appear, we can use cell salts to fill our reserves, and if we have a chronic condition, we must do so quite slowly to replace our deep-well reserves. Once our mineral needs are met, we can be healthy, strong, energetic, mentally clear, and at peace with others and ourselves.

Using the twelve basic cell salts, we can counterbalance many deficiencies and cure or avoid diseases and other health conditions. Prevention is always important. Although we may feel well now, pollution, stress, etc., tax our mineral reserves. Those of us who are taking macro and trace minerals may still have deficiencies and may not be obtaining the physical, mental, and spiritual benefits we seek from them. For instance, gastrointestinal challenges may reduce our ability to absorb the minerals. Stomach problems, indigestion, gas, etc., are signs of poor mineral absorption. Cell salts, by their preparation, are reduced to a size small enough to be easily assimilated into the cellular structure of the body, hence the name cell salts. (Other books refer to them as tissue salts, as they are derived from minerals important for the body's tissues.) Acid blockers or other medications also restrict our ability to absorb minerals. This is another reason to use cell salts! I recommend taking cell salts until your local and deep mineral reservoirs have been replenished, which is evident when your health and vitality have been restored, and then continue to use them for another 2–3 months.

Dr. Carey and Inez Eudora Perry have also provided metaphysical explanations of the cell salts in their book *Cell Salts of Salvation*, in which they make correlations between the twelve cell salts and the twelve astrological constellations, a practice common amongst many medieval- and Renaissance-era doctors. You can see a symbolic rendering of their views on page 9. In this rather esoteric book, the authors suggest that each of us has a "birthday" cell salt (determined by the sign of the zodiac under which we were born) that we should take on a regular basis to support our health.

USE AND HANDLING OF CELL SALTS

1. Liquid – Take the number of drops indicated on the bottle, unless otherwise directed. Place drops directly under the tongue and retain for at least 30 seconds. Avoid touching the mouth or tongue with the dropper.

2. Pellets – Avoid touching pellets with hands. Put desired number of pellets into lid of container and drop them into the mouth. Let them dissolve under the tongue; do not chew or swallow them. Pellets can also be placed in water – preferably distilled. Add them to the water, stir, and then sip throughout the day.

3. Topical applications – The topical application of cell salts sends the minerals directly to the affected area for fast and effective results. Topical cell salt applications are very simple. One can crush the pellets between two spoons and sprinkle the correct cell salts on the skin area. (The recommendations for topical applications of various cell salts will be found in the chapters that follow.)

   Another method of topical application involves putting 10 pellets of each recommended cell salt into a pint of hot or cold water (as required for the individual case) and stirring the water with a non-metallic spoon until the cell salt is dissolved. Then, soak a cloth in this treated water, wring out the cloth, and apply it to the affected area until there is relief, or until another application is required. You may choose to put another dry cloth over the soaked cloth to protect your outer clothes or the bed sheets.

   One can also crush the cell salts (10 pellets) and put into one ounce of a neutral-based (non-medicated or non-perfumed) cream or lotion (a moisturizing cream can also be used). Apply the lotion or cream to the affected area. This form delivers the salts in a slower but longer lasting application.

4. Do not brush teeth, eat, or drink anything (except for water) for at least 10 minutes before or after administering the remedy.

5. Keep all cell salt remedies out of direct sunlight. Do not store them near a microwave oven, computer, or television set. Do not

store them near substances with strong odors such as essential oils. It is not necessary to refrigerate them.

6. Do not use any gum, mints, or toothpaste containing peppermint or spearmint within 30 minutes of taking the remedy. It is important to refrain from using any products containing camphor of menthol while under treatment. These products can antidote the remedies.

7. Caffeine, especially coffee, can reverse the action of cell salts. However, decaffeinated coffee, either instant or freeze-dried, does not appear to antidote the remedies.

8. Do not allow cell salts to pass through airport x-ray scanners. Either pack them in a lead-lined photo bag in checked baggage or request that they be hand-inspected by security personnel. Passenger walk-through devices are okay.

9. When the directions given suggest alternating one remedy with another, switch remedies every 2–4 hours. In acute situations, alter remedies every few minutes.

10. Sometimes when taking a particular remedy, the healing process stalls. In some situations the recommendation is to take another remedy "intercurrently." In this case one would stop taking the first remedy, take the second remedy until there is a shift, and then return to the first remedy.

11. Throughout this book you will notice references to using different cell salts at different points in the healing process (e.g., "first remedy," "second stage of resolution," "third remedy.") There are three stages in the course of any disease or condition. The first relates to inflammation; the second, to infection or discharge of pus; and the third, to resolution (the body gets rid of the pus). Different cell salts are suited to addressing different stages in this process.

12. Cell salts come in a variety of potencies. The most commonly used are the "6x" potencies, that are found in most health food stores. If there is an emergency or one cannot find this exact potency, use what you have. Potencies can vary from 3x to 200x, or 6c to1000c, and beyond. The lower potencies – 6x to 30x – are within the scope of the use for this book. Higher potencies require expertise or a consultation with a homeopath (a doctor or health practitioner who recommends the use of homeopathic remedies and cell salts). The 6x to 30x potencies can work miracles. I recommend having all twelve cell salts on hand. The various individual cell salts and combinations can serve to promote better health, not previously realizable. If you can't find cell salts in your local health store, consult the sources listed in the back of this book.

FACIAL DIAGNOSIS

Facial diagnosis for cell salt deficiencies was pioneered by Dr. Schuessler (1821–1898) and was verified and expanded by Dr. Hickethier (1891–1958). Various practitioners in Germany such as doctors, homeopaths, and pharmacists have done further work in this area. (See Bibliography.) Very little has been written on this topic in English. I have started to disseminate this material in English and hope that the English-speaking world will catch on to this simple way to detect cell salt deficiencies.

I have used this method of diagnosis successfully for fifteen years and my clients have been very satisfied. They have only seen greater health and success. I hope that each family will use this book to prevent diseases and treat minor maladies. I believe professionals will recognize that cell salts can be easily used in their practice as an adjunct to other therapies or as a stand-alone to promote health. The great thing is that you cannot make mistakes with cell salts, as they are non-toxic and safe to take regardless of age, gender, physical condition (including pregnancy and nursing), or current medication regime.

FACIAL LOCATIONS THAT INDICATE CELL SALT DEFICIENCIES

The photo on page 5 indicates the places to look for signs of cell salt deficiency. In the list that follows, next to each cell salt you will find the major facial location or locations where a deficiency of this salt can be observed. For example, a deficiency of the salt **Calc Fluor** is easily observed around the eye sockets (see photo on page 5), the tips of the teeth, or the lips. For a more detailed explanation of the deficiency indicators mentioned below, please refer to the relevant cell salt chapter.

CALC FLUOR – around the eye sockets, translucent tips of teeth, cracked lips.

CALC PHOS – ears, nose, skin under eyebrows, cheekbone, small lips, translucent tips of teeth.

CALC SUPLH – jaw line.

FERRUM PHOS – *chronic*: whole-face paleness, bluish-black circles under eyes; *acute*: red cheek, forehead, ears.

KALI MUR – cheeks, eyelids.

KALI PHOS – sunken temples and cheeks, overall gray coloring, dull eyes.

KALI SULPH – brown to yellow entire face, typically around the mouth.

MAG PHOS – general facial redness or acute blushing.

NAT MUR – lower eyelashes, nose, cheek, chin or forehead.

NAT PHOS – general yellow to red coloring: nose, mouth, forehead, chin, and cheeks.

NAT SULPH – general green coloring to a chronic red; indications on the nose; bags under the eyes.

SILICEA – bald head, shiny nose, wrinkles that start by the ears, sunken eyes, crow's-feet wrinkles.

FACIAL SKIN APPEARANCE INDICATING CELL SALT DEFICIENCIES

This listing is an overview of the major cell-salt-deficiency indicators (Shine, Color and Texture) that are observable in the facial skin. This list indicates which cell salt best remedies each condition. For example, with a **shiny face** that appears **greasy**, you would use the salt **Nat Phos**. For a more detailed explanation of the deficiency indicators mentioned below, please refer to the relevant cell salt chapter.

SHINE

CALC FLUOR – Reflective, especially in acute conditions.

NAT PHOS – Greasy. It has a greasy feel.

NAT MUR – Gelatinous. This is often found on the upper eyelid or the edge of the eyelashes on the lower eyelid. When the greasy part of the skin is wiped clean, this quality will reappear after 20-30 minutes.

SILICEA – Glassy or polished.

COLOR

CALC FLUOR – Blue lips, brownish-black shading, white flakes, transparent tips of teeth.

CALC PHOS – White waxy appearance, transparent tips of teeth.

CALC SULPH – Alabaster-white appearance, paleness.

FERRUM PHOS – Bluish-black shade, red ears.

KALI MUR – Milky red, or blue, or purple shading; acne rosacea; red spider veins.

KALI PHOS – Ash-gray.

KALI SULPH – Brownish-yellow or ocher pigmentation, liver spots, age spots, vitiligo, freckles.

MAG PHOS –Redness (chronic).

NAT MUR – Red border at hairline.

NAT PHOS – Red chin.

NAT SULPH – Greenish-yellow, bluish-red, yellowish.

SILICEA – No special color

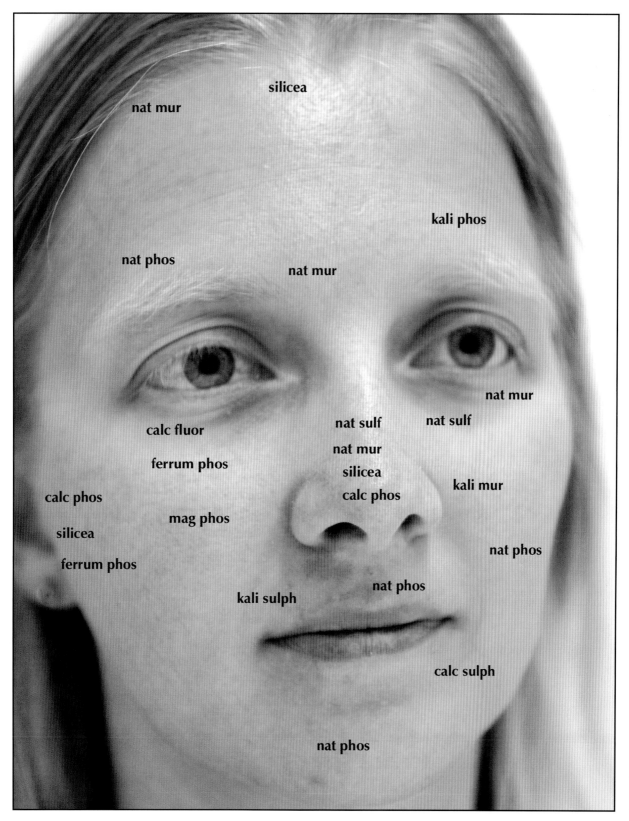

This photo indicates where you would see specific cell salt deficiencies on the face.

TEXTURE

CALC FLUOR – Raised wrinkles, fan-shaped wrinkles, furrows, white scales, cracked lips, translucent tips of teeth.

CALC PHOS – Waxy appearance, white flakes in teeth or fingernails, translucent tips of teeth, stretched skin on cheekbones, small lips.

FERRUM PHOS – Shading in corners of the eyes, furrows, hung-over or sleepless appearance, red ears, inflamed skin.

KALI MUR – Milky appearance, acne rosacea, chicken skin.

KALI PHOS – Ash-gray appearance, frosted look of eyes, sunken cheeks, bad breath.

KALI SULPH – Brownish-yellow appearance, pigmentation, freckles, vitiligo, pregnancy mask, brown spots.

MAG PHOS – Chronic redness, acute blushing, alcohol redness.

NAT MUR – Inflamed eyelids, large pores, dandruff, dry skin, puffy cheeks, spongy or bloated appearance, bell-shaped nose, sweaty or greasy skin.

NAT PHOS – Combination skin, cholesterol deposits (raised yellow pimple-like growths around the eyes), blackheads, pimples, acne, upper lip wrinkles, fatty deposits, red chin, acid spots, dry skin, dry or greasy hair, greasy sweat.

NAT SULPH – Greenish-yellowish coloring, swollen lower eyelid sacks, yellowish sclera, bad-smelling gas.

SILICEA – Wrinkles in general, vertical wrinkles parallel to the ears, laugh lines, crow's feet, deep-set eyes, split ends, sensitivity to light, fingernail problems, red eyes (burst veins of the eyeballs).

Cell Salt Astrology

At the end of each chapter I have included Dr. Carey's correlations between the cell salts and the planets/astrology. This may interest you if you study astrology. Even if you don't, you may still appreciate the connections between the cell salts and the months of the year. Dr. Carey noted that many people have been benefited by using their "birth cell salt," the one designated for the time period during which they were born.

That is just one of many ways to take cell salts. Another possibility is to use them in a cyclical fashion, that is, take each one throughout its assigned month, rotating to a new cell salt each new astrological month. In simple terms, there is a time and a season for everything. The cell salts are no different. Over the course of a year, this progression allows you to cleanse, purify, and strengthen the body.

Explanation of the Illustration: Symbols of Alchemy, Astrology and Cell Salts

The illustration on page 9, by the wonderful artist Monique Ordonez, is based on an ancient yet timeless concept of the Philosophical Egg. The illustration represents several levels of symbolism concerning natural life cycles. It derives from Dr. Carey's work and also from ancient alchemical knowledge. Good references on this subject include: *The Cell Salts of Salvation* by Carey, *The Practical Handbook of Plant Alchemy* by Manfred M. Junius, and *Culpeper's Medicine* by Graeme Tobyn.

The natural cycles represented in this illustration are described briefly below.

The Elements

One way of looking at the world is by dividing everything into four parts. In this schemata, one of four elements (earth, air, fire, water) is associated with every constellation and planet.

The elements thus divide the universe into four parts and correspond to the four directions, the four seasons, and the human's four constitutions (or "humors"). The humors are blood, phlegm, choler, and melancholic. Graeme Tobyn explains them very well. The **fire** element represents heat, fire, and dryness. The properties of the corresponding planet, constellation, etc., show these qualities. This element is represented by an upturned triangle.

The **air** element is representative of damp and warm conditions. It is represented by an upturned triangle with a horizontal bar.

The **earth** element is cold and dry and is represented by a down-turned triangle with a horizontal bar.

The **water** element is wet and cold and is represented by a down-turned triangle.

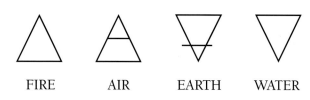

FIRE   AIR   EARTH   WATER

The Constellations

The constellations are time representations that have been linked to organs, systems, seasons, etc. The constellations are another way to look at month-like periods. The ancients were able to track the "months" according to astronomical indications, and they named these constellations. Each constellation has its own story. Associations with stories were a way to make the seasons come alive. People then remembered how to order their lives according to celestial time and thus had a closer connection to the seasons.

The constellations divided the year and the universe into twelve parts. Twelve is a very sacred number common in many cultures.

The Planets

The planets were considered "travelers in the sky." This is why the ancients also included the sun and moon as travelers. The planets were symbols of the "sacred seven" used by most cultures throughout the ages.

These planets in the sky were the closest celestial objects to earth, so they were known to affect us most closely. Planets were considered to be more influential than the constellations.

The planets shown in this illustration govern the constellations. This means that planets and constellations have an influence on each other, although there is not always a direct organ correlation between the constellations and planets. The "planets" concept of health is explained in depth in my book *Seven Symbols of Healing and Testing*.

The Seasons

Healthcare professionals have noticed that the seasons affect our health and the health of our organs. The ancients noticed this too. This illustration shows the progression of the seasons as associated with the organs, cell salts, etc.

Progression of Time

The illustration shows a seasonal progression of time as shown by the arrows; this is part of the continual change and predictability of life.

Alchemy

There is an alchemical process (like dissolution, distillation, or fermentation) associated with each of the constellations as suggested by Manfred M. Junius in his book *Practical Handbook of Plant Alchemy*. All are processes of purification. They also imply possible symbolic interpretations when associated with the cell salts, times, seasons, etc. These processes are:

Aries – calcination, a process of burning away impurities to a very refined state.

Taurus – congelation, whereby cold changes the structure for purification.

Gemini – fixation, a process of stabilization to create perfection.

Cancer – dissolution, which involves putting one substance into another to create better health.

Leo – digestion, thus separating good from bad substances.

Virgo – distillation, or creating heat to separate and purify.

Libra – sublimation, which means immersing one's self, or bringing a separation.

Scorpio – separation, which takes things apart to purify them.

Sagittarius – incineration, which burns away the dregs of one's impurities.

Capricorn – fermentation, creates a separation by creating a more pure product and toxin release.

Aquarius – multiplication, brings on a separation process to bring more possibilities.

Pisces – projection, showing our vulnerability and possible cleansing

The Snake

The symbol of the snake represents the ancient concept of "Ouroboros," or "One Eternal Round." This may also represent the wedding band, where there is no beginning and no end. This snake symbol also shows a cleansing process brought about by taking the cell salts as a cleansing system throughout the year. This is a continuing symbol as is our constant attention to purification and the perfection of our inner self.

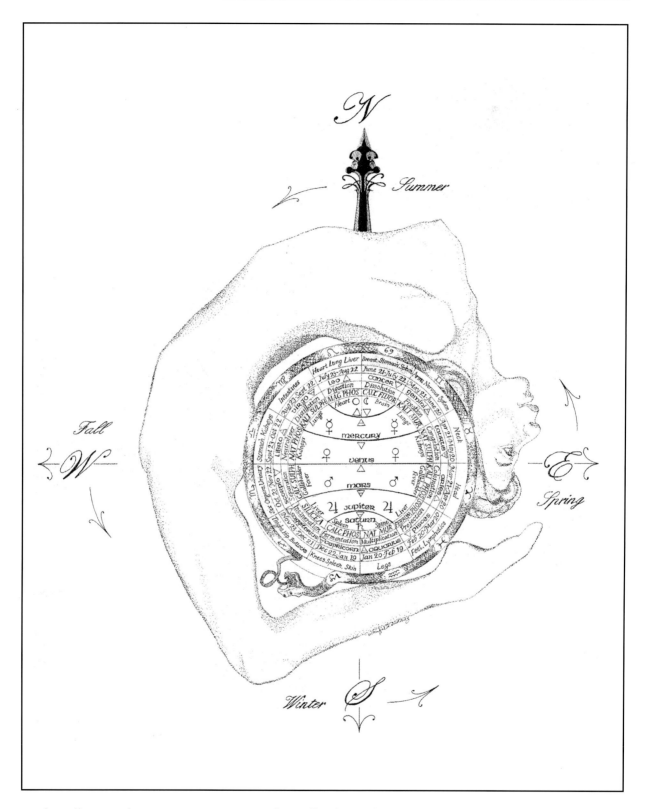

This allegorical representation pairs the cell salts with the Zodiac signs and seasons, thus indicating which cell salts would be used when, to cleanse and purify the body. Posters of this diagram are available; see page 170.

CHAPTER 2

Introduction and History

Biochemistry, or biochemic treatment of disease, opens up a new phase of medical science. The treatment of disease, with the inorganic cell salts is so rational, so in accordance with well-known principles of natural law, that its basic principles need only be presented to the intellect to be understood and adopted.*

The original communication by Schuessler to the German journal was translated into English by Dr. H. C. G. Luyties, and soon afterwards appeared in a small edition by Dr. C. Hering, on the twelve biochemic remedies.

Later, Doctors Boerick and Dewey published a book, *The Twelve Tissue Remedies*. It was the following words of Professor Moleschott of Rome, in his work *Vital Circulation*, which set Schuessler to thinking that the sick might be healed with "substances that are natural, i.e., physiological function remedies."

On this fact is based the high estimation, in which of late years, the subject of the relative proportions of the inorganic (mineral) substances to the individual parts of the body has been held.

In the face of such positive facts, it can no longer be denied that the substances which remain after incineration or combustion of the tissues – the ashes – are as important and essential to the inner composition, and consequently to the "form-giving" and "kind-determining" basis of the tissues, as those substances that are changed during combustion.

A connective base and bone-earth are essential constituents of bone. Without either there can be no true bone; so also, there can be no cartilage without cartilage salt, nor blood without iron, nor salines without potassium chloride (Kali Mur).

The word "biochemistry" is formed from "bios" (the Greek for "life") and "chemistry." Webster defines chemistry as "that branch of science

*This complete introductory section is adapted from:
The Biochemic System of Medicine by Dr. George Carey.

which treats the composition of substances and the changes which they undergo." Therefore, biochemistry, taken literally, means that branch of science which treats the composition of living substances, both animal and vegetable, and the processes of their formation. But usage has given the word somewhat different signification, and the following is a more accurate definition: *That branch of science which treats the composition of the bodies of animals and vegetables, the processes by which the various fluids and tissues are formed, the nature and causes of the abnormal condition called disease, and the restoration of health by supplying to the body the deficient cell salts.*

The chemical composition of nearly every fluid and tissue in the human body has long been known, but until biochemistry was introduced, no practical use had been made of this knowledge in the treatment of the sick. Biochemistry is the only system of medicine which answers satisfactorily and fully the question: "What is disease?" It not only does this, but it gives a logical reason for every dose of cell salt prescribed and describes its action in the system.

Biochemistry is science, not experimentalism. There is no more mystery and miracle about it than about all natural laws. The food and drink taken into the stomach and the air breathed into the lungs furnish all the materials of which the body is composed. By the juices of the stomach, pancreas, and liver, the food is digested and the useful particles are taken by the villi of the small intestines. These are carried by the blood to the various parts of the body where they are needed and where they are absorbed. The blood thus supplies the materials necessary for forming every tissue and fluid in the body and for carrying forward every process.

An analysis of the blood shows it to contain organic and inorganic matter. The organic constituents are sugar, fat, and albuminous (egg-white-like protein) substances. The inorganic constituents are water and certain minerals, commonly called cell salts. Of a living human being, water constitutes over seven-tenths; the cell salts, about one-twentieth; organic matter, the remainder.

Not until recently were the inorganic cell salts understood and appreciated. Being little in quantity, they were thought to be lesser in importance. But now it is known that the cell salts are the vital portion of the body, the workers, the builders; that the water and organic substances are simply inert matter used by these salts in building the cells of the body.

Should a deficiency occur in one or more of these workers, of whom there are twelve, some abnormal condition arises. These abnormal conditions are known by the general term "disease," and as they manifest themselves in different ways and in different parts of the body, they have been designated by various names. But these names totally fail to express the real trouble. Every disease which afflicts the human race is due to a lack of one or more of these inorganic workers. Every pain or unpleasant sensation indicates a lack of some inorganic constituent of the blood. Health and strength can be maintained only so long as the system is properly supplied with these cell salts.

Man, through the medium of plant life, is a product of the soil. All the main elements enter into his composition. Were the soil barren of its constituent matters, plant life would be unknown and man would cease to exist. An equilibrium of the inorganic constituents is as necessary in fertile soil and plant life as in the human organism. It is a law immutable and has existed since the world's creation.

Having learned that disease is not a thing, animate or inanimate, but a condition due to a lack of some inorganic constituent of the system, it follows naturally that the proper method of cure is to supply to the system that which is lacking. While in the treatment of disease, the use of products not constituents of the system may be very necessary and useful, a complete return to health cannot be expected until the missing cell salts are supplied.

Biochemistry would seek to ascertain what is lacking and supply it in just the form needed. Any disturbance in the molecular motion of these cell salts in living tissues constituting disease can be rectified and the requisite equilibrium reestablished by administering the same mineral salts in small quantities. This is brought about by virtue of the operation of chemical affinity in the domain of histology, and hence this therapeutic procedure is styled by Schuessler as "the Biochemic Method," and stress is laid on the fact that it is in harmony with well-known facts and laws in physiological chemistry and allied sciences.

It is the blood that contains the material for every tissue of the body, that supplies nutriment to every organ, enabling it to perform its individual function; it is, indeed, a microcosm, able to supply every possible want to the physical body.

Two kinds of substances are needed in the process of tissue building, and both are found in the blood, namely the organic and inorganic constituents.

DISEASE – NATURE'S EFFORTS TO RESTORE EQUILIBRIUM

Adapted from: *Chemistry of the Cosmos*, by Dr. George Carey

Disease is an alarm signal, a friend that calls to inform us of danger. Disease is an effort to prevent death. Therefore, pain and so-called "disease" is more than a warning; it is an effort that opposes death. The symptoms that indicate disease are calls, or dispatches, asking for the material with which repair of bodily tissue may be made. Pains or discomforts of various functions or structures of the body are words asking for the constituent parts of blood, nerve fluids, tissue, bone, etc.

If acids cause pain, the pain is a call for a sufficient amount of alkaline salts to balance an acid effect and change fluids to a balanced and natural state. Healthy synovial fluid (fluid of the joints – the lubricator) is neither acid nor alkali but yet contains both in combination. Should the alkaline salts become deficient in amount for any cause, the acid at once becomes a disturbing element and hurts the nerves that pervade the membranes of periosteum (bone covering) of the internal structure of knee, elbow, or other joints of the human anatomy. This pain, or word, cannot be considered bad or malignant in any sense.

So then it matters not what name may be given to nature's demand for reinforcements through the medium of pain or any symptom that indicates a deviation from the plane of health; one thing and one thing alone is needed, i.e., to supply the blood with the dynamic molecules, the twelve cell salts, that set up vibration or action in the human machine.

Poisons, of whatever name or nature, do not and cannot supply deficiencies and cure disease for the simple reason that poisons are not constituent parts of the human organism.

Poisons oppose calls for help and tend to still the voice of nature; therefore, the effect of poison is towards death. Many have survived the effects of poisons, but equally many have been hurried to their graves.

A proper use of mineral or cell salts of the blood in the potency and proportion found in the ashes of a cremated body will do all that can be done medicinally to supply deficiencies and restore normal conditions.

The cell salts form the chemical base of the blood, and blood builds all tissue and fluids of the body.

Anarchy is increasing. A lot of people even refuse to be poisoned by vaccine pus, and some have declared their intention to select their own mode of treatment when sick. Now it is up to the lawmakers to "stamp out such anarchistic doctrine."

All phenomena is a result of Divine, beneficent law, hence disease so-called is the result of the orderly procedures of that law. In all ages all men and women have been sick more or less. In all ages there have been storms, cataclysm, earthquakes, and extremes of heat and cold; no one questions the wisdom that causes, guides, and directs these events, then why should we question the wisdom of disease? Disease is one phase of the transmutation of matter in the procedure of regeneration.

All methods of healing are phases of the transmutation process

"THE CLINICAL EVIDENCE OF THE TRUTH OF SCHUESSLER'S INDICATIONS IS OVERWHELMING AND SINCE HIS TIME THEY HAVE BEEN LARGELY CONFIRMED BY HOMEOPATHIC AND ECLECTIC PHYSICIANS."

– WILLIAM BOERICKE, M.D., AND W.A. DEWEY, M.D.

"THE BODY IS A SELF-CURING MECHANISM, AND IT WILL MAINTAIN ITS EFFICIENCY PROVIDED IT HAS A NORMAL SUPPLY OF ALL THOSE ELEMENTS PARTICULAR TO ITS OWN SUBSTANCE."

– ERIC POWELL, PH.D, N.D.

ORGANS AND TISSUES AFFECTED BY CELL SALT DEFICIENCIES
(compilation by David R. Card)

CALC FLUOR – Connective tissue, bones, vein walls, tendons, sinews, tooth enamel, throat, **larynx, thyroid.**

CALC PHOS – Bones, muscles, teeth, spine, blood, periosteum (bone covering), cartilage, glands.

CALC SULPH – Liver, gallbladder, heart muscle, connective tissue, glands, mucus membranes, bones, skin.

FERRUM PHOS – Blood, arterial system, colon, lungs, Eustachian tubes, heart, mucus membranes, bones.

KALI MUR – Glands, bronchials, throat, Eustachian tubes, ears, muscles, joints.

KALI PHOS – Spleen, nerves, muscles, mucus membranes, skin.

KALI SULPH – Pancreas, liver, skin, mucus membranes, glands, respiratory organs.

MAG PHOS – Heart, colon, nerves, muscles.

NAT MUR – Kidneys, blood, mucus membranes, cartilage, brain, heart, spleen, liver.

NAT PHOS – Stomach, tissues, lymphatics, genitals, intestines.

NAT SULPH – Liver, gallbladder, pancreas, colon.

SILICEA – Connective tissue, skin, nerves, hair, nails, glands, bones, Eustachian tubes, cartilage.

PHYSICAL SYMPTOMS OF CELL SALT DEFICIENCIES

(compilation by David R. Card)

CALC FLUOR – Cornea problems, chapping, cracking skin, cavities, varicose veins, osteoporosis, deficient teeth enamel.

CALC PHOS – Osteoporosis, nosebleeds, bone growth, late teeth, heart palpitations, nose polyps, headaches (in children), growing pains.

CALC SULPH – Chronic pus, open infections, fibroids, yellow mucus discharges, boils.

FERRUM PHOS – First stages of fever (99–101°), pulsing and throbbing headaches, inflammations, anemia, hemorrhages, sore throat, nosebleeds, colds, flus.

KALI MUR – Second stages of fever (101–103°), coughing, Eustachian tube blockage, white mucus discharges.

KALI PHOS – Bad breath, nerve and sleep problems.

KALI SULPH – Third stage of fever (103–105°), cravings for fresh air, skin dandruff, thick yellow discharges, constantly changing symptoms.

MAG PHOS – Chocolate cravings, blushing, cramping and shooting pains, muscle paralysis.

NAT MUR – Head cold and congestion; clear, watery discharges; sun sensitivity; cold sores.

NAT PHOS – Acne, blackheads, greasy or brittle hair, split ends, over acidic conditions.

NAT SULPH –Foul-smelling gas, swollen feet or hands, head injuries. Worse in wet, cold or damp weather.

SILICEA – Light sensitivity, hip pains, fragile skin, scarring, hernia, sweaty hands and feet.

FOODS RICH IN CELL SALT NUTRIENTS

(compilation by David R. Card)

CALC FLUOR – Whole grain foods, dairy foods, raw vegetables, soybeans, sesame seeds, spinach, broccoli, mushrooms.

CALC PHOS – Almonds, cucumbers, oats, soybeans, white beans, dandelions, cherries, spinach, dairy foods, dates.

CALC SULPH – Oats, almonds, cucumbers, lentils, peanuts, soybeans, cauliflower.

FERRUM PHOS – Spinach, hazelnuts, whole rice, soy, sesame seeds, tomatoes, oats, red and blue berries.

KALI MUR – Cucumber, peanuts, hazelnuts, lentils, spinach, pork, soybeans, sesame seeds, potatoes.

KALI PHOS – White beans, soybeans, cucumbers, almonds, spinach, pork, hazelnuts, peanuts, lentils.

KALI SULPH – Pork, hazelnuts, peanuts, almonds, spinach, lentils, peas, nuts.

MAG PHOS – Brazil nuts, white beans, wheat, soybeans, corn, walnuts, peanuts, peas.

NAT MUR – Red beets, lentils, radishes, tomatoes, sea salt, milk, celery, celery seeds, goat whey.

NAT PHOS – Lentils, pork, asparagus, spinach, rose hips, oats, olives, carrots.

NAT SULPH – Lentils, pork, spinach, oats.

SILICEA – Millet, whole rice, oats, whole grains, wheat, peas, carrots, cucumbers, strawberries, parsley.

EMOTIONAL SYMPTOMS OF CELL SALT DEFICIENCIES
(compilation by David R. Card)

CALC FLUOR – Indecisiveness, weakness, low self-esteem, stress regarding financial matters.

CALC PHOS – Desire to travel, loss of motivation, mental weakness, difficulty handling bad news.

CALC SULPH – Fatigue, laziness, inactivity, worries about imaginary problems.

FERRUM PHOS – At first, stimulation and overheating, followed by dullness and listlessness.

KALI MUR – Family issues, irritability, apathy, homesickness, tendency to hypochondria.

KALI PHOS – Nervous irritability, weak memory, test anxiety, tension, moody depression, anger, self-pity, feeling of being insulted and disgraced by family.

KALI SULF – Fearful dreams, need for self-validation, sensitivity to noises, irritability, anger.

MAG PHOS – Sensitivity, outgoing nature, complaints regarding physical problems, impulsivity, quick action.

NAT MUR – Isolation, control issues, sun sensitivity, deep grief, forgiveness issues.

NAT PHOS – Depression from overly sensitive nerves, sleeplessness, low self-esteem.

NAT SULPH – Depression from wet weather or head injuries.

SILICEA – Shyness, lack of "grit," hypersensitivity, sensitivity to cold.

Note: Emotional symptoms from mineral deficiencies may or may not be present. They often show up in cases of deep or chronic deficiency.

TONGUE SYMPTOMS OF CELL SALT DEFICIENCIES
(compilation by David R. Card)

CALC FLUOR – Tongue is cracked, inflammation, and swelling, hardness, can be painful or not.

CALC PHOS – Bitter taste in mouth with blister or pimples on the tip of the tongue, the tongue is swollen, stiff and numb.

CALC SULPH – Inflammation, infected sores. Flabby with yellow coating at back.

FERR PHOS – Red to dark red with inflammation and swelling with no coating.

KALI MUR – Tongue can be coated grayish-white, dry or slimy.

KALI PHOS – Coated dark yellow to brown, dry and inflamed and swollen. "Creeping paralysis."

KALI SULPH – Coated yellow and slimy with a dull taste in mouth.

MAG PHOS – Swollen clean tongue (a swollen tongue usually has teeth marks on the edge).

NAT MUR – Frothy coating, bubbles on the sides. Numbness and tingling. Peeled appearance on sides.

NAT PHOS – Yellow creamy coating on back of tongue. Blisters on the tip with stinging; hairlike sensation on tongue.

NAT SULPH – Greenish-brown swelling or gray coating on the back of tongue or slimy thick white mucus coating.

SILICEA – One-sided swelling of tongue. Brown tongue, hardening and ulcered. Sensation as if a hair on tongue.

DISCHARGES INDICATIVE OF CELL SALT DEFICIENCIES
(compilation by David R. Card)

CALC FLUOR – Grass-green discharges or thick yellow-greenish discharges, that smell offensive.

CALC PHOS – Thick clear discharges.

CALC SULPH – Yellow thick and lumpy discharges.

FERR PHOS – Hemorrhages of blood from inflammatory conditions anywhere in the body.

KALI MUR – Thick white discharges.

KALI PHOS – Profuse orange discharges from rectum or vagina. Yellowish creamy discharges in general.

KALI SULPH – General yellow to green slimy discharges. Profuse and thin discharges.

MAG PHOS – White thin discharges of the nose and dark stringy vaginal discharges.

NAT MUR – Clear thin watery discharges

NAT PHOS – Sour, creamy or honey colored thin discharges.

NAT SULPH – Watery yellowish to greenish discharges.

SILICEA – Thick yellow offensive discharges from boils and infections, and sweating. Infected parts are often painful.

Note: These discharges can come from any part of the body.

* * *

Discharges show us the condition of our immune system. When the body produces **mucus**, it is trying to clear the body of toxins.

Clear discharges show a clearing of the body or the beginning of a cold, flu, allergy, or a hormonal condition.

White discharges are a sign of mucus congestion.

Yellow discharges are less serious if the color is getting lighter, but can be worse if it gets darker.

Green discharges are signs of infection.

Brown discharges are serious infected conditions.

Black discharges indicate the worst condition, which is indicative of dried blood. See a doctor.

CHAPTER 3

Calc Fluor

The inorganic salts are the workers, controlled and directed by Infinite Intelligence, which perform the ceaseless miracle of creation or formation.*

It is quite as important for a student of biochemistry to understand the process by which certain cell salts operate to supply a deficiency as it is to know for what a particular symptom calls.

Elastic fiber, the chief organic substance in rubber, is formed by a chemical union of Calc Fluor, also known as calcium fluoride, with protein, oil, etc. Therefore we find this salt dominant in the elastic fiber of the body, in the enamel of teeth and connective tissue. A lack of this salt in proper amount causes a relaxed condition of muscular tissue, falling of the womb, and varicose veins. Sometimes there is a nonfunctional combination of this salt with oil and protein, which forms a solid deposit, causing swelling of stony hardness. A combination of impure substances corrupts the chemistry of calcium fluoride to create a hardening of the tissues.

There is one particular symptom that is worthy of note in connection with the pathology of this salt. When a deficiency exists in these makers of elastic fiber in the connective tissue between the cerebellum and cerebrum, the lower and upper brain, it causes groundless fears of financial ruin. It seems that the relaxed condition of connective tissue, causing a sagging of the structure of cerebellum, thereby breaks the flow of the electrical or magnetic currents from the cerebrum.

The student will now see that it is exceedingly easy to diagnose disease from the viewpoint of biochemic pathology. No guesswork here. Go to twenty or one hundred biochemic physicians and give the same symptoms to each, and you will get the same prescriptions in every case.

It does not matter under what name a disease a disturbance in elastic fiber appears, a study of the chemistry of life has made clear the fact that a

*This complete introductory section is adapted from:
The Chemistry and Wonders of the Human Body by Dr. George Carey.

break in the molecular chain of Calc Fluor salt is always the cause of the phenomenon.

The proportion of fluorine in the human organism is less than that of iron. From analytical facts is found that fluorine in milk is only present in micrograms, and yet we are confronted by the fact that this infinitesimal amount is sufficient to sustain all the elastic fiber of muscular tissue, enamel of teeth, and connective tissue.

Why should we search Latin and Greek lexicons to find a name for the result of a deficiency in some of the mineral constituents of blood? When we know that deficiency in the cell salts of the blood causes the symptoms which medical ignorance dignified and personified with names of which nobody knows the meaning, we will know how to scientifically heal by the unalterable law of the chemistry of life. When we learn the cause of disease, then and not before, will we prevent disease.

MATERIA MEDICA FOR CALC FLUOR

Adapted from: *The Biochemic System of Medicine, Materia Medica*, by Dr. George Carey

This salt occurs in nature as the mineral fluorspar, beautifully crystallized, of various colors, in lead veins, the crystals having commonly the cubic but sometimes the octahedral form, parallel to the faces of which latter figure they always cleave. Some varieties, when heated, emit a greenish and some a purple phosphorescent light. The fluoride is quite insoluble in water but is decomposed by sulphuric acid, generating hydrofluoric acid.

Calc Fluor (calcium fluoride) is found in the surface of the bones, the enamel of the teeth, the elastic fibers, and the cells of the skin. Wherever elastic fiber is found, be it in the epidermis, the connective tissue, or the walls of the blood vessels, there calcium fluoride may always be found. Loss of its ability to unite with organic matter causes a continued dilation or relaxed condition

of the fibers. This is seen in such conditions as varicose veins, hemorrhoidal tumors, and relaxation of the abdominal walls, with consequent sagging of the abdominal viscera, uterine hemorrhages, after-pains, etc.

This state of relaxation, occurring in the elastic fibers of the blood vessels, connective tissue, or lymphatic system causes an inability to absorb discharges. This results in hardened glands, lumpy discharges on the surface of bone, encysted tumors, hard swellings, etc. By supplying the lacking Calc Fluor, the elastic fibers are again restored to their integrity, resuming their power of contractility and functioning properly. Discharges are thrown off and absorbed by the lymphatics.

In general, then, the administration of Calc Fluor is indicated in all diseases which can be traced, directly or indirectly, to relaxed conditions of the elastic fibers or those ailments having their seat in either the substance forming the surface of bone, enamel of the teeth, and walls of the blood vessels or the cells of the epidermis.

Characteristic Indications

(Note: **Remedies in parentheses provide therapeutic support to Calc Fluor.**)

Head – Troubles with head when traced to a relaxed condition of the elastic fibers. Tumors on the heads of newborn infants, blood clots. Bruises on the bones of the head, when they have hard, rough, uneven lumps. Ulcerations of the bone surface.

Eyes – Cataracts. Blurred vision after straining the eyes, with pain in the eyeball; better when resting the eyes, as relaxation of the walls of the blood vessels allows for an engorgement of blood.

Ears – Diseases of the ear, when the bone or periosteum (bone covering) is affected, or with general symptoms characteristic of this salt.

Nose – Stuffy cold in the head, with thick, yellow, lumpy, greenish, foul-smelling nasal discharge, also known as ozena (Kali Phos, Silicea).

Diseases of the nose, when affecting the bones (Calc Phos).

Face – Hard swelling on the cheek, with pain or toothache. Bony lumps or growths on the jaw or cheekbones.

Mouth – Cracked lips (Nat Mur); very hard swellings on the jawbones, traceable to the relaxed condition of the muscular fibers.

Teeth – Teeth become loose in their sockets, not during dentition, with or without pain. The enamel of the teeth is largely composed of this salt. Enamel rough and thin or very brittle. Rapid tooth decay when the enamel is deficient (Calc Phos). Teeth tender due to looseness.

Tongue – Cracked appearance, becomes hard after inflammation (Silicea). Chronic swelling of the tongue.

Throat – Relaxed condition of the throat. Elongation of the uvula (fleshy mass of tissue suspended from the center of the soft palate), causing tickling cough as it drops into the throat (Nat Phos). Diphtheria, when the disease has entered the windpipe (Calc Phos). Enlargement of the throat (Nat Mur). Relaxation of the blood vessels of the throat.

Gastric symptoms – Vomiting of undigested food. Ferrum Phos is the principle remedy for this condition, but when this fails, use Calc Fluor.

Abdomen and stool – Hemorrhoids, when bleeding. Protruding and itching hemorrhoids, blind hemorrhoids, accompanied with pain in back and constipation. Alternate with remedies indicated by color of stools or blood (see page 2, for topical applications). Also apply remedy locally. Hemorrhoids with rush of blood to the head (also requires Ferrum Phos); confined bowels; inability to expel the feces due to a relaxed condition of the rectum, allowing too much fecal matter to accumulate. This condition occurs frequently in the 4–6 weeks after childbirth, when all the pelvic muscles are relaxed. Anal fissure, sore crack near end of bowel; should also apply remedy locally in this case.

Urinary organs – Increased quantity of urine, when traced to a relaxed condition of the muscular fibers in the urinary organs.

Male sexual organs – Swelling or hardening of the testicles. In cases of syphilis, when other symptoms indicate this remedy.

Female sexual organs – All displacements of the uterus (uterine prolapse) require this remedy (Calc Phos, Kali Phos). Falling of the womb. Anteversion (tipped uterus), retroversion (bending backwards of the uterus), and flexions of the uterus require this salt to tone up the contractile muscles. Dragging pains in the groin and in the lower part of the back; pains extend to the thighs. Menses excessive, hemorrhaging, with bearing-down pains. Uterus very relaxed and flabby, or very hard like stone, due to the disorganization of the fluoride of lime molecules.

Pregnancy – After-pains, when too weak. Hemorrhage, if the uterus does not contract. Hard knots and lumps in the breast (Kali Mur).

Respiratory organs – Uvula (fleshy mass of tissue suspended from the center of the soft palate) elongated, causing tickling in larynx, with cough. Cough, when tiny lumps of tough, yellow mucus are expectorated (Silicea). In asthma, when the expectoration is difficult and consists of small, yellow lumps (Kali Phos). Improvement when patient is relaxed and lying down.

Circulatory organs – Varicose veins, with a tendency for this condition. Veins seem as if they might burst; apply lotion containing the salt as well. Dilation of the blood vessels when the elastic fibers of the walls of the vessels have become relaxed; Calc Fluor is the chief remedy to restore their contractility (Calc Phos). First stage of aneurysm (Ferrum Phos). Hypertrophy, or enlargement of the heart (Kali Mur). Irregularities of the heart's action, when due to prolapse of uterus and other diseases related to excessive relaxation.

Back and extremities – Pain in lower part of the back, weak, with dragging pains. Burning pains in the sacrum, with confined bowels. Hard growths or excrescences on the bone surface (scoliosis). Relaxed conditions of the muscles, also discoloration of the fingers and toes. Hard swellings. Gouty enlargement of the joints (Mag Phos). Varicose ulceration of the veins of the limbs; apply lotion containing the salt using cotton. Cover legs with a poultice of Calc Fluor, Silicea, and Calc Sulph.

Skin – Hangnails. Hands or lips chapped from cold (Ferrum Phos). Skin hard or horny; also use plenty of soap and water. Cracks in the palms of the hands; mix a quantity of the cell salt in Vaseline, and after washing the hands, rub the ointment in thoroughly. Anal fissures, fistulous ulcers, when secreting thick, yellow pus (Silicea, Calc Sulph).

Tissues – Pus or infections of the bones and periosteum (bone covering), ulcers, felons (infected hangnails). "When a fibrinous [of fibrous protein] discharge is not dissolved by suppuration [discharge of pus from infection], but has become hardened, Calc Fluor must be given" (Schuessler). Encysted tumors, swellings, hardened enlargements, hardened glands, etc. (Kali Mur, Silicea). Relaxed elastic tissues. Bone bruises, with uneven hard lumps. Swelling or water retention from heart disease.

Febrile conditions – Fevers, when arising from relaxed conditions. To address the cause of these fevers, alternate Calc Fluor usage with these remedies: Ferrum Phos, first; Kali Mur, second; Kali Sulph, third.

Modalities – Heat will generally give relief, especially for hardened conditions; cold is sometimes beneficial when contraction is required.

FACIAL SIGNS OF CALC FLUOR DEFICIENCY

Cubic-shaped raised lines appear in a cross-hatched pattern, starting from the inner corner of the eye and expanding outward across the lower or upper eyelid. Note: The finer the lines, the greater the cell salt deficiency.

Diamond-shaped raised lines start on the inner corner of the eye and proceed in a sloping or curving fashion across the lower or upper eyelid. They look like parallelograms or rhombuses. Within these, one can see small raised points. In acute cases the lines have a fine or stretched appearance, and in chronic cases the wrinkles look deeper, appearing like a hanging sack. Note: It is easier to examine these patterns when the patient's eyes are closed.

Fan-shaped wrinkles start at the inner corner of the lower part of the eye. Have the person close their eyes tightly in order to see these.

Brownish-black coloring, though it is often hard to perceive. This is a brown with black undertones. The more intense the color, the greater deficiency.

Blue lips show there is a strong Calc Fluor deficiency, as the muscle and artery strength has been compromised and the heart is having to work harder. (We also see blue lips with a combined deficiency in Nat Sulph and Ferrum Phos.)

Reflective shine, one of three shines that appear when there are cell salt deficiencies. In this case the skin is as clear as glass or water, with a very thin lacquered appearance. This comes not from the stretched skin, but from a fine layer of keratin on the skin which reflects light.

Small white scales can be a sign of significant Calc Fluor deficiency; in this case the keratin layer is flaking off. Referred to as the fish-scale disease, this often appears on the upper eyelid. Note: This is an indirect sign of a Calc Fluor deficiency, so use other signs to verify.

Cracked lips, especially in cold weather. Note: This is an indirect sign of Calc Fluor deficiency, so use other signs to verify.

Translucent tips of teeth can be a sign of a Calc Fluor, as well as a Calc Phos, deficiency. With a deficiency in Calc Fluor, a patient may also lack enamel on the teeth.

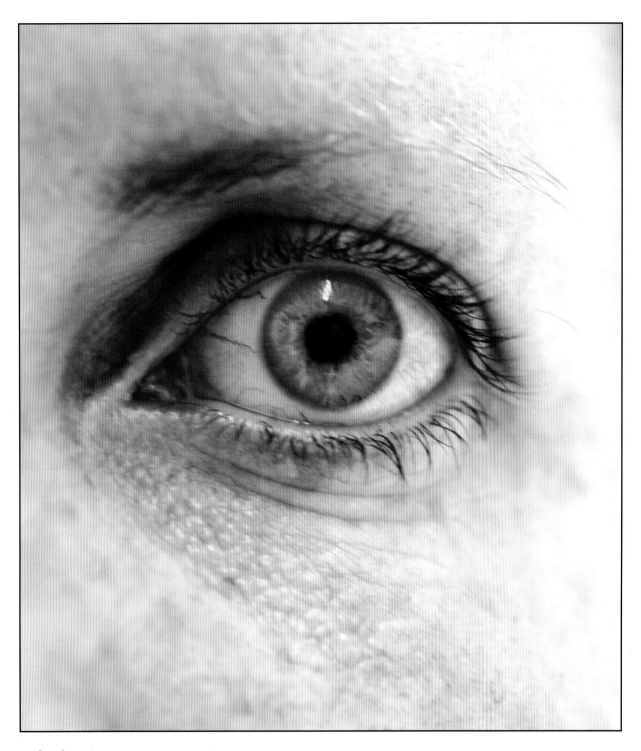

Calc Fluor (a)

The close-up of this eye shows a typical Calc Fluor raised wrinkle in the corner of the eye, and the brownish-black circle under the eye. The eye has the deep-set Silicea look. The waxy coloring around the eyes shows a Calc Phos deficiency. This waxiness covers an underlying red layer of skin; the red layer shows a Mag Phos deficiency. The half eyebrow is a possible indication of a hypothyroid condition.

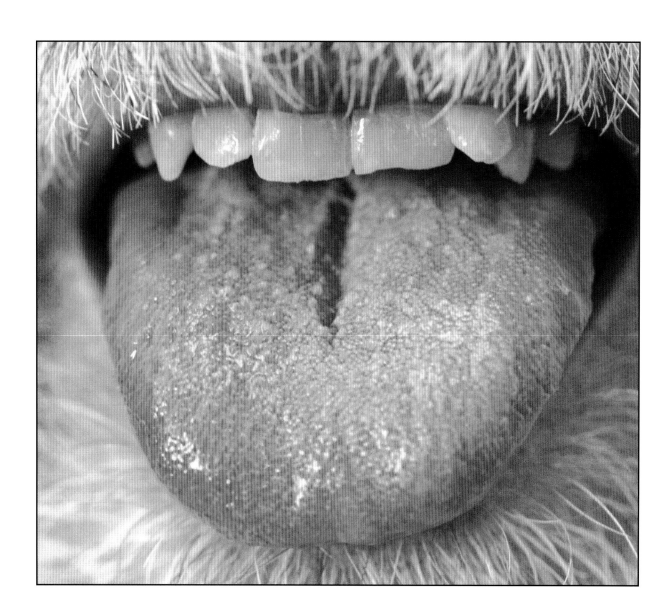

Calc Fluor (b)

This man's teeth are very translucent, characteristic of a Calc Fluor deficiency. The tongue pimples are a sign of a Nat Phos deficiency and possible overgrowth of candida in the body.

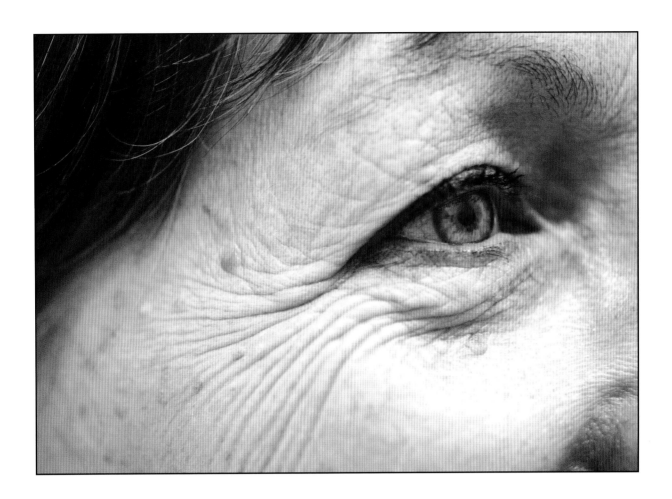

Calc Fluor (c)

This picture shows a severe Calc Fluor deficiency with the fan-shaped crow's feet. There is a waxy Calc Phos deficiency noticeable above the eyes. The bag under the lower eye indicates a Nat Sulph deficiency and can be a sign of a kidney or liver problem.

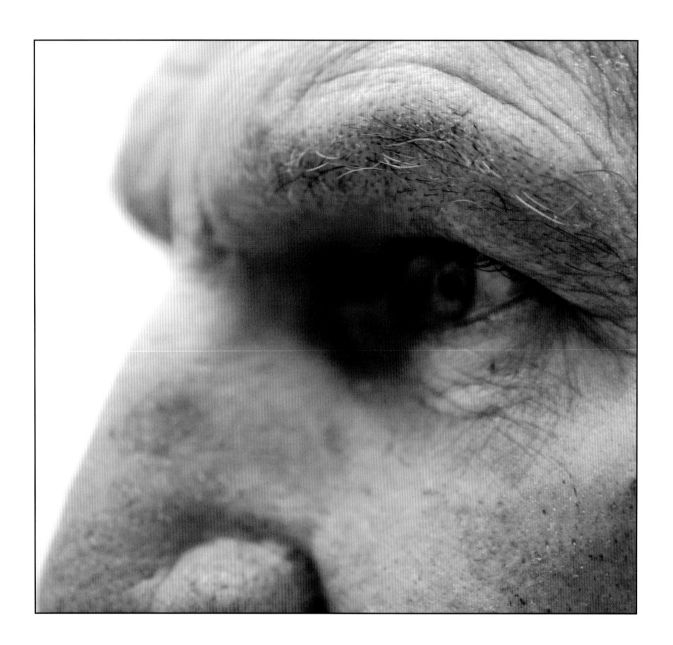

Calc Fluor (d)

The brownish-black circle under this eye exemplifies a Calc Fluor deficiency. This man also has a Silicea deficiency, indicated by his deep-set eyes. He also has a liver problem, and this yellowish-brown liver sign can be addressed by using Kali Sulph.

Calc Fluor Summary

ORGAN AND TISSUE AFFINITIES
Bones, veins, tooth enamel, tendons, sinews, glands, elastic fiber, periosteum (bone covering), throat, larynx, binding of tissues, elasticity of tissues.

MODALITIES
Symptoms worse < cold, wet, change of weather, damp weather, sprains, beginning motion.
Symptoms better > by continued motion, heat, applications of heat, rubbing.

DEFICIENCY SYMPTOMS
Brittle, splitting, soft nails; cracking skin; low body temperature; sweaty feet.

DISEASE CONDITIONS
Bone problems, cataracts, tooth enamel problems, hardening glands, gas, tumors, weak connective tissue, scoliosis, scar tissue, splinters, smelly feet.

THERAPEUTIC INDEX OF CALC FLUOR
Adapted from: *Therapeutic Index* [1890] by Dr. W. H. Schuessler

Cephalhematoma (blood clots in the brain).
Cornea, opacities, spots on the.
Enamel of teeth deficient.
Exudations on the bone surface; hard, rugged (corrugated), pointed elevations.
Knots, hard, of the female breasts.
Ozeana (foul-smelling nasal discharge). See also Calc Phos.
Suppuration (discharge of pus from infection) of the bone.

Swellings, hard, having their seat in the fascia and capsular ligaments.
Swellings of the jaw.
Testicles, induration (hardening) of.

ASTROLOGY OF CALC FLUOR
Cancer: The Chemistry of the Crab
June 21 to July 22
Adapted from: *Cell Salts of Salvation* by Dr. George Carey

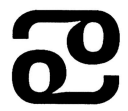

Cancer is the Mother Sign of the zodiac. The mother's breast is the ego's first home after taking on flesh and "rending the Veil of Isis." The tenacity of those born between the dates June 21 and July 22 in holding on to a home or dwelling place is well illustrated by the crab's grip, and also by the fact that it carries its house along wherever it goes in order that it may be sure of a dwelling.

The angels of the twelve zodiacal signs materialize their vitalities in the human microcosm. Through the operation of chemistry, energy creating the intelligent molecules of Divine Substance makes the "Word" flesh. The cornerstone in the chemistry of the crab is the inorganic salt fluoride of lime, known in pharmacy language as Calcarea Fluorica. It is a combination of fluorine and lime. When this cell salt is deficient in the blood, physical and mental disease (not at ease) is the result.

Elastic fiber is formed by the union of the fluoride of lime with albuminoids (egg-white-like proteins), whether in the rubber tree or the human body. All relaxed conditions of tissue (varicose veins and kindred ailments) are due to a lack of sufficient amount of elastic fiber to "rubberize" the tissue and hold it in place. When elastic fiber is deficient in the membrane tissue between the upper and lower brain poles

– cerebrum and cerebellum – there results a "sagging apart" of the positive and negative poles of the dynamo that runs the body's machinery. An unfailing sign or symptom of this deficiency is a groundless fear of financial ruin. While those born in any of the twelve signs may sometimes be deficient in Calc Fluor, Cancer individuals are more likely to manifest symptoms, indicating their lack of this elastic fiber-builder.

The governing planet of this water sign is the Moon. The gems associated with Cancer are black onyx and emerald, and the colors are green and russet brown. In Bible alchemy (an esoteric interpretation of the Bible), Cancer is represented by Zebulum, the tenth son of Jacob, whose name means "dwelling place" or "habitation." Matthew is the New Testament disciple associated with this sign.

CHAPTER 4

Calc Phos

As bone is the foundation of the animal structure, I will commence with the bone builder – Calc Phos, also known as calcium phosphate. Bone tissue is about 57 percent calcium phosphate. The calcium salt has chemical affinity for protein. While there is a certain degree of affinity between each of the cell salts and protein – protein being the base of all organic matter – the operation of calcium phosphate with protein is greatest. The salt chemically unites with protein, carries it, and uses it as cement to build bone tissue. Bone also contains carbonate of soda, magnesium phosphate, and sodium chloride, but calcium phosphate is the chief builder of bone tissue, and it follows, as a logical sequence, that it is the principal salt deficient in all so-called diseases of bone structure.*

The gelatin found in bone tissue is formed by the union of protein, oil, carbon, calcium, and phosphate in certain proportion. A lack in the proper amount of this builder, in some instances, causes an anemic condition, for bone material (calcium and protein) is the foundation of bodily structure.

Under certain conditions, dependent on deficiencies in other cell salts, a break in the molecular chain of calcium phosphate will cause an outflow of protein through the kidneys. Why should the escape of albumen (egg-white-like protein; also referred to as "albuminoids") through the kidneys be named Bright's disease? It seems that the fact of the loss of albumen in this manner was first discovered in the case of a hospital patient named Bright, and although many others die in a regular and orthodox manner from the same cause that cut off the immortal Bright, the medical profession has dignified the disease by the original label. The very same albumen that causes Bright's disease, if expelled through the nasal passage, is called catarrh (mucus congestion), from the Greek word meaning "to drop down."

If albumen reaches the skin, by disintegration or fermentation it causes pimples, eruptions, eczema, etc. If anyone derives pleasure from these

*This complete introductory section is adapted from:
The Chemistry and Wonders of the Human Body by Dr. George Carey.

names, well and good, let them use them, but chemistry knows nothing whatever about them.

A great deficiency in Calc Phos may cause protein to accumulate in some gland and there disintegrate and flow out in pus, or heteroplasm (dissimilar tissue), which is called scrofula (swelling of the lymph nodes) by the old-school physicians.

The calcium molecules are found in the fluids of digestion and assimilation, and when there is a lack of the proper amount of these workers, the digestive juices become negative, lose their proper rate of motion or catalytic action, ferment, and thus produce gas, acid condition, etc. When calcium phosphate and sodium phosphate – the alkaline salts – are deficient, acids, together with albuminous substance, may settle in the joints and thus render synovial fluids "nonfunctional," thereby causing pain, stiffness, and swelling of the joints. Just why this chemical fact must needs have the word "rheumatism" tacked to it does not appear. The word "rheumatism" is derived from the word "rheum," meaning "to flow out."

MATERIA MEDICA FOR CALC PHOS

Adapted from: The Biochemic System of Medicine, Materia Medica by Dr. George Carey

Calc Phos (also known as phosphate of lime or calcium phosphate) is destined to play a prominent part in the treatment of the sick when its range is fully understood by medical practitioners. This salt works with albumen, carrying it to the bone, tissue, or any other part of the body where it may be needed. It uses albumen as a cement to build up bone structure.

Bone is 57 percent phosphate of calcium, the remainder gelatin (an albuminous, gluey substance), carbonate of soda, magnesium phosphate, and sodium chloride. Without the calcium (Calc Phos), no bone can be made.

When, for any reason, the molecules of this salt fall below the proper standard in the blood,

a disturbance occurs in life's processes. It may be that bone cells are not rebuilt as fast as they die. In such cases, if the deficiency exists for a great length of time, a condition of anemia prevails, for the bone is the basis, the foundation stone, of the organism. Should the albumen, not having a sufficient quantity of the Calc Phos to properly take care of it, become a disturbing element and be thrown off via the kidneys, Bright's disease results. If through the nasal passages, the condition is named catarrh (mucus congestion). If by the lungs, a cough is produced. If the albumen reaches the skin, pimples, eruptions, freckles, a condition called eczema, or possibly sores result.

Calcium phosphate is found in gastric juice, and a lack thereof is frequently the cause of indigestion.

Conditions called rheumatism are sometimes due to a deficiency of this cell salt. It is well known to biochemists that a proper balance of sodium phosphate (Nat Phos) is required to prevent an acid condition from prevailing, and under certain conditions, when calcium phosphate for any reason is not present in proper quantities, the affinities draw upon sodium phosphate in an endeavor to supply the lack, and thus a deficiency in that alkaline salt ensue, which allows an acid condition to prevail, i.e., rheumatism. Calcium phosphate is also an auxiliary to the therapeutic effects of magnesium phosphate, as it more nearly resembles that salt than any other. When Mag Phos is clearly indicated and it does not restore the normal condition in a reasonable length of time, Calc Phos should be given, for it is quite certain that it has been drawn on from the blood to assist the work of Mag Phos, hence the deficiency in the calcium salt.

Characteristic Indications

(Note: Remedies in parentheses provide therapeutic support to Calc Phos.)

Mental – Peevishness and fretfulness in children. Poor memory, incapacity for concentrated thought, mind wanders from one subject to another, weak minds in those practicing or who have practiced masturbation (Kali Phos). Dullness, stupidity, depression of spirits, anxiety about the future. Desire for solitude after grief (Nat Mur), disappointment, pain, etc.

Head – Headache, with cold feeling in the head, also head feels cold to the touch. Headache on top of head and behind the ears. Tight sensation. Headache in girls during puberty, with restlessness and nervousness. **Headache worse from mental exertion, worse near the cranial sutures. Skull thin and soft. Closure of the fontanelles delayed, or reopening of same.** Vertigo (Ferrum Phos). **Crawling, cold sensations over the head.** Ulcers on top of head. Dropsy (swelling) of the brain. Loss of hair; bald spots. Inability to hold up the head. (Nat Mur)

Ears – Aching pain, with swelling of the glands of face and neck. Earache with characteristic clear, thick, excoriating (irritating) discharge. In scrofulous (those with lymphatic swelling) persons, where the glands are very swollen. Ears swollen, burning, and itching.

Eyes – Sensitivity to artificial light. Eyeballs ache; spasm of the eyelids (Mag Phos). Squinting. Hot feeling in the eyelids. Paralysis of the retina, causing dimness and loss of sight (Kali Phos). Neuralgic pain in eyes, when Mag Phos fails. Inflammation of the eye, with characteristic discharge, especially in scrofulous subjects. Light sensitivity (Ferrum Phos, Nat Mur).

Nose – Large, pedunculated (on a stalk) nasal polyps. Nose swollen (from congestion) and greatly inflamed at the edges of nostrils (Silicea). Tip of nose cold. Congestion, cold in head. Thick, clear, tough discharge, dropping from posterior nares, causing constant hawking and spitting; worse outdoors. In anemic persons, disposition to take cold (Ferrum Phos). Preparing the way for other remedies in all cases of catarrh, Calc Phos has a decided tonic action on the membranes.

Face – Anemic or chlorotic (greenish tint to skin) face. Dirty-looking face. Rheumatism of the face, which is worse at night. Pimples on the face. Facial pains, with a creeping sensation; feeling of coldness and numbness. Face sallow, pale, earthy; skin cold and clammy. Lupus. Heat in face. Freckles, eruptions on the faces of young persons, especially of young girls at puberty. Facial pains, of a grinding, tearing nature (Mag Phos). Pale face in children, when teething is difficult.

Mouth – Unpleasant, disgusting taste in mouth in the morning caused by non-assimilation of food (Nat Phos).

Teeth – Retarded dentition (Calc Fluor). Phosphate of lime (Calc Phos) is a constituent of the teeth, and when this material is deficient, dentition will be slow and painful, often causing convulsions (Mag Phos) and other ailments. Teeth decay as soon as they appear. Gums inflamed and painful (Ferrum Phos). Toothache, which is worse at night (Silicea). **Chief remedy in all teething disorders.** "If the gums be pale, this remedy is especially indicated" (Schuessler).

Tongue – Swollen tongue (Kali Mur). Stiff and numb. Blisters and pimples on tip of the tongue.

Throat – Enlargement of the throat. Chief remedy for goiter (Nat Mur). **Chronic enlargement of the tonsils.** "I have given it in the acute stage, when suffocation threatened, with excellent results," (Chapman, [see: full reference to Chapman's book in the Bibliography]). Glands painful, aching. Thirst, with dry tongue and mouth. **Sticking pain in throat on swallowing.** Constant hoarseness. Hemming and scraping of throat when talking. (Public speakers are greatly benefited by this cell salt when alternated with Ferrum Phos.) Burning and soreness in larynx and pharynx, in cases of chronic catarrh when there is considerable dripping from the posterior nares (postnasal drip).

Gastric symptoms – Pain after eating. **Food seems to lie in stomach in a lump.** Heaviness and burning. Pain worse from eating even the smallest amount of food (Ferrum Phos). Stomach sore to the touch. Abnormally large appetite, but food causes distress. Cold drinks and food greatly aggravate the pains, while heat relieves it (Mag Phos). **Vomiting after cold drinks.** Faint, sinking feeling in region of stomach. Pain sometimes relieved by belching wind. In infants, vomiting sour, curdled milk (Nat Phos). Constant desire to nurse. Stomach feels bloated. Headache, accompanied with indigestion (digestive headache). Belching of gas. Most of these gastric symptoms are due to non-assimilation of food. A course of this remedy should be given after gastric or typhoid fever and in all cases where digestion is poor to aid assimilation of food.

Abdomen and stool – Diarrhea in teething children; stools slimy, green, with undigested matter; with colic (Nat Phos). Give a warmwater enema. **Cholera infantum,** child craves food it should not eat. **Stool is hot, noisy, and offensive-smelling** (Kali Phos). Inability to properly digest food during the summer. Diarrhea caused from inability to properly digest food. Face pale and anxious, child fretful. Pain in the abdomen near the navel. Infant cries when it nurses. Marasmus (failure to thrive), eats heartily but grows more emaciated all the time. **Frequent urge to pass stool but nothing passes** (Kali Phos, Mag Phos). Diarrhea in young girls, with accompanying headache. Costiveness (constipation), with hard stool, in old people and infants. Itching piles, also protruding hemorrhoids (Calc Fluor, Ferrum Phos). Hemorrhoids, which ooze a thick, clear substance resembling egg whites, especially noticeable in anemic persons. **Anal fissures and cracks** (Calc Fluor). Fistula without pain. Neuralgia of rectum and pain after stool. **Symptoms all worse at night or with change in**

weather (Silicea). Tabes mesenterica (abdominal lymph-wasting disease). To prevent the formation of gallstones.

Urinary organs – Urine dark yellow. Frequent urge to urinate, with sharp, shooting, cutting pains at the neck of the bladder and along the urethra (Ferrum Phos). Increase in the quantity of urine. Bright's disease of the kidneys (Kali Phos). Phosphatic deposit in the urine, as an intercurrent remedy. Gravel sediment in urine (Nat Sulph). Diabetes mellitus, as an intercurrent remedy. To prevent formation of bladder stones. Calc Phos assists in the breaking down of protein that can accumulate in the kidneys.

Male sexual organs – Swelling of the testicles (orchitis). Masturbation. Inguinal (groin area) hernia (Calc Fluor). Itchy, greatly relaxed scrotum. Sweating and soreness of scrotum. Chronic gonorrhea and gleet (chronic inflammation of a bodily orifice), when there is the characteristic discharge. Swelling of the testicles. Egg-white-like discharges from the urethra.

Female sexual organs – **Weakness in uterine region from prolapsed uterus and other uterine displacements** (Calc Fluor, Kali Phos). "Calc Phos may not have the contracting power of Calc Fluor, by acting directly upon the muscles and tissues involved, but it acts indirectly by building up the general health and aiding digestion, thereby restoring the tissues to a healthy condition and promoting the deposit of Calc Fluor" (Chapman). **Aching** in the uterus. Increased sexual desire, especially immediately before menstruation. Leucorrhea (white discharge from the vagina), with thick, clear, very tenacious discharge. Intercurrently in all cases of leucorrhea, to build up general health. Acrid leucorrhea, worse after menstruation or with sexual excitement. Dullness and listlessness. In young girls with anemic conditions, menses too early or too late. Menstrual discharge bright red, too frequent. Menses with pain in back. Laborlike pains at the time of menstruation (Mag

Phos); to prevent, use Ferrum Phos. Menses, with flushed face and cold extremities (Ferrum Phos).

Pregnancy – Aching in the limbs during pregnancy. Poor milk, watery or with salty taste (Nat Mur). Child refuses to nurse. Child vomits sour, curdled milk quite frequently. Sore nipples (Ferrum Phos). **After pregnancy**, as a restorative; also **after long nursing**, when the patient is debilitated.

Respiratory organs – Cough, with expectoration of clear (not yellow), thick mucus. Chronic coughing. Incipient consumption (tuberculosis). Intercurrently in all cases for weakness and prostration. Chronic cases of whooping cough. **Rheumatic pains in lungs. Involuntary sighing.** Soreness and dryness of tuberculosis in throat. Aching in the chest. Night sweats, especially around the head (Silicea, Nat Mur). Hawking to clear throat. Cough in anemic persons or teething children.

Circulatory organs – Intercurrently in most cases of heart trouble. Poor circulation, with cold extremities. Palpitation of the heart, followed by weakness. Leukemia (excess of white corpuscles in the blood).

Back and extremities – Calc Phos, appropriately named "the bone remedy," plays an important role in disease located in the back and extremities. Curvature of the spine (Scoliosis). **Numbness and coldness** of the limbs. Pains and aching in the joints. **Cold sensations in the limbs, as if cold water were being poured over them.** Pains in the bones, especially the shinbones. Pain worse at night and in cold, damp weather. **Rheumatism of the joints and in the back between the shoulders; very severe and worse at night or during rest.** Lumbago (Ferrum Phos). Hydroma patella (swelling of the knee caps), cysts. Hydrops (swelling). Articular (joint) spinal irritation. Injuries of the coccyx. Infants are slow in learning to walk, and their bones are soft and friable.

Bowlegs (used in conjunction with mechanical supports). In children, thin neck (Nat Mur). Broken bones; this salt is essential to facilitate the deposit of extra material necessary for their mending. Rickets: "This disease appears to consist essentially in the nondeposition of phosphate of lime in the osteoid (bone) tissues" (from *Thomas' Medical Dictionary*, as cited by Dr. Carey. In the case of syphilis, inflammation of the periosteum (bone covering). Ulcers and abscesses, when deep-seated on the bones or joints. Neuralgia, when deep-seated as if on the bone, commencing at night (Silicea). Pain in limbs, restlessness, limbs fall asleep; better when moving them.

Nervous symptoms – **Neuralgia**, which is worse at night, colic, cramps, spasms, convulsions, etc. (take if Mag Phos fails to relieve these symptoms). Convulsions in teething children, young girls, and old people, when the calcium salts are deficient. Paralysis, when associated with rheumatism. Fatigue and weariness. **Pains very severe at night, with sensation of creeping numbness and coldness. Pains shoot all over the body like electrical shocks and, at other times, like trickling cold water.**

Skin – Eruptions on the skin, when the discharge is thick and clear. Pimples, acute or chronic, with itching. Itchy skin, without eruptions. Eczema, with yellowish-white crust. Face full of pimples. Scrofulous affections, intercurrently. Dry skin. Skin itching and burning, as from nettles. Perspiration on hands from spinal weakness. Lupus, with characteristic symptoms. Pruritus (itching) of vagina, with or without thick, clear leucorrhea (Nat Mur). Freckles (apply a 10 percent solution of cell salt in water to the face). Chafed skin (Nat Mur). Acne rosacea. Tubercles (nodules) on the skin. Scaly herpes on the shins.

Tissues – Bones weak, easily broken; when broken, bones will not unite or, when new bone material is needed. Rickets. Tabes, or atrophy of

Calc Phos Summary

ORGAN AND TISSUE AFFINITIES

Nutrition, **bones**, tendons, teeth, protein muscles, cartilage, chest.

MODALITIES

Symptoms worse < teething, loss of fluids, exposure to cold, wet wind, thinking of symptoms, puberty, eating fruit, night.

Symptoms better > summer warmth, dry weather, lying down, rest.

DEFICIENCY SYMPTOMS

Muscles are sensitive to cold. White marks on fingernails and teeth. Tips of teeth are translucent.

DISEASE CONDITIONS

Bone problems, weak ankles, teething problems, osteoporosis, spina bifida, stiff neck, rickets.

any organ tissue. Poor nutrition through indigestion. Ulceration of bone substance. Stunted growth. Defective development, with pale, greenish-white complexion. Polyps. Disease of the pancreas. Emaciation, chlorosis, anemia. Intercurrently in all bone affections, constitutional weakness. As a tonic for delicate, anemic persons (Ferrum Phos). All ailments caused by a deficiency or disturbance in the phosphate of lime (Calc Phos) molecules.

Febrile conditions – Chilliness and shivering, when beginning of fever (Ferrum Phos). Excessive perspiration, **night sweats in cases of phtisis (known as tuberculosis)**. **Cold, clammy sweat on the face and body**. After typhoid and other fevers, as the disease recedes, to promote the deposit of new material in place of that destroyed.

Sleep – Restless sleep due to worms (Nat Phos), drowsiness, sleepiness, difficulty waking in the morning. Vivid dreams.

Modalities – Symptoms are generally **worse at night in damp, cold weather** (Nat Sulph), with change of weather, upon getting wet, etc. **Better in warm weather and in warm room.**

FACIAL SIGNS OF CALC PHOS DEFICIENCY

A **waxy appearance** is often seen on areas with cartilage such as the nose, ears, etc. The more facial surface having this waxy quality, the greater the deficiency.

Ears may appear waxy on the cartilage and ear muscle. Look for a waxy intensity.

Eyebrows Look for a waxy appearance to the skin. There may also be waxy-looking stripes coming diagonally from the eyebrows.

White spots on the teeth and nails show a Calc Phos deficiency. We also see teeth with translucent tips (Calc Fluor).

Stretched cheekbone musculature is another sign. People with this symptom exhibit a biting or hard-bitten look or character, as though life has dealt them a hard hand.

Small lips also suggest a hard life. These signify poor mineral absorption.

Yogurt appearance, a creamy-whitish look. This can occur in the case of Calc Sulph deficiency as well.

THERAPEUTIC INDEX OF CALC PHOS

Adapted from: *Therapeutic Index* (1890) by Dr. W. H. Schuessler

Anemia, first remedy
Bone diseases, see also **Rickets**.

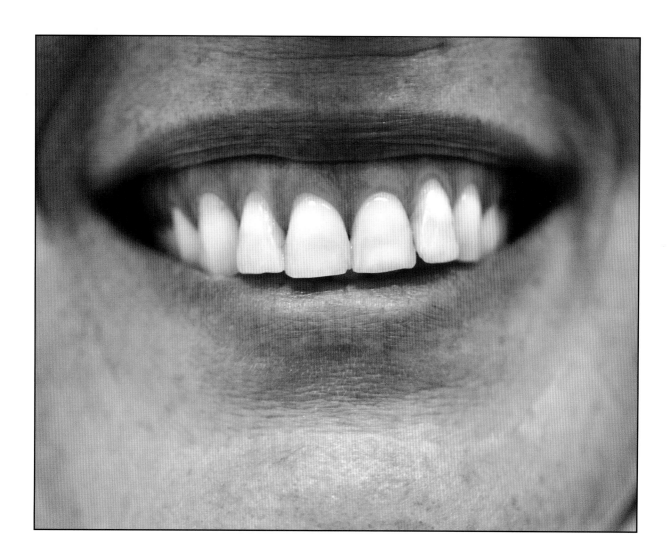

Calc Phos (a)

The tips of the teeth clearly show the translucent quality of a Calc Phos deficiency. A Calc Fluor deficiency can also show up as translucence of the teeth. The chin is red and thus shows a Nat Phos deficiency. There are brownish spots on the skin that show a Kali Sulph deficiency.

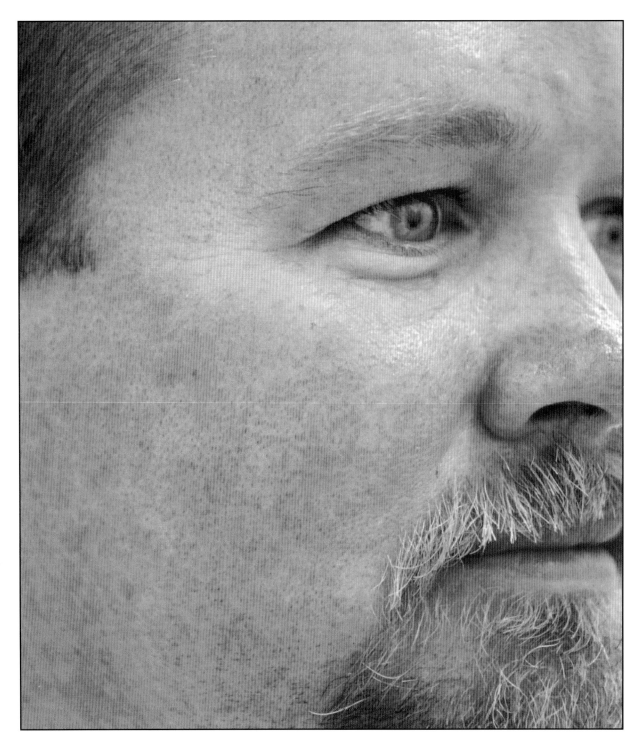

Calc Phos (b)

This picture shows a Calc Phos deficiency with a waxy appearance around the eyes, root of the nose and into the eyebrows. The redness of the cheeks shows a Kali Mur deficiency.

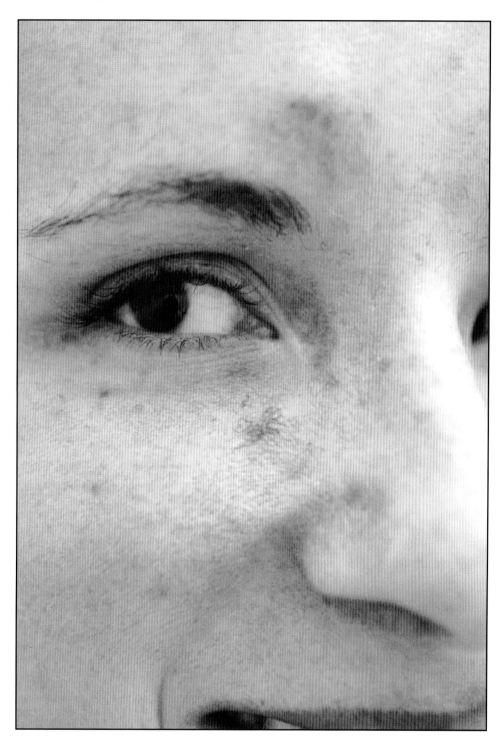

Calc Phos (c)

This woman shows a Calc Phos deficiency by the waxy appearance around her eyes, nose and forehead. She also has a Nat Phos deficiency because of the appearance of the red acne blemishes. The brownish-black of the inner eye area is a Calc Fluor deficiency sign. The middle of her forehead has a greenish tinge, suggestive of a Nat Sulph deficiency.

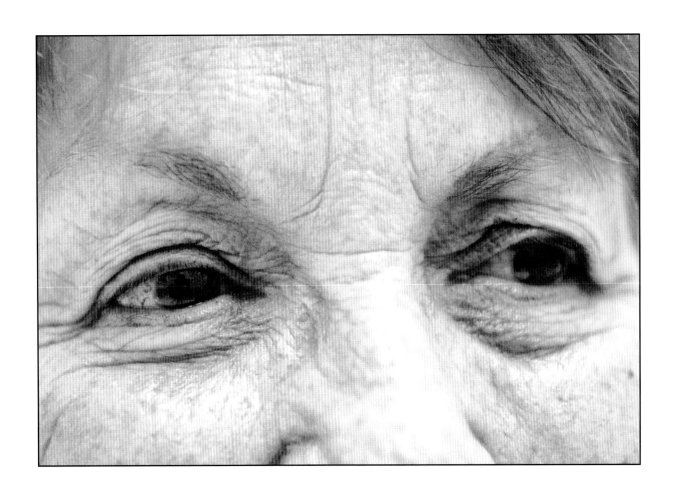

Calc Phos (d)

This woman has the Calc Phos deficiency symptoms of a waxy appearance of the root of the nose, eyes and into the eyebrows. She has the reddish overlay indicative of a Mag Phos deficiency, and a Calc Fluor deficiency can be noted in the raised pattern in the corner of the eyes. The bags under her eyes denote a Nat Sulph deficiency. Her squinting appearance, horizontal lines on the root of the nose, and short eyebrows also show a hypothyroid condition. Such conditions accompany a weak liver. Another sign of liver malfunction is seen in the greenish appearance, a Nat Sulph deficiency.

Cancer, in scrofulous (swelling of the lymph nodes) constitutions.

Catarrh (mucus congestion), in chronic or anemic persons.

Chlorosis (greenish tint to skin) type of anemia.

Convalescence, during and after acute diseases.

Convulsions, from teething, without fever, if Mag Phos fails.

Cough, in consumption (tuberculosis).

Delicacy, in growing girls and children.

Diabetes mellitus.

Diptheria, first remedy, to reduce the fever and limit inflammation of throat.

Dropsy (swelling), from non-assimilation or anemia.

Eczema, with anemia.

Eczema, with dry, crusty affections.

Enuresis (urinary incontinence), nocturnal, from general weakness.

Eyelids, spasmodic affection, if Mag Phos fails.

Face ache (neuralgic, rheumatic), worse at night.

Fits (epileptic), during development in childhood and youth.

Fits, in the scrofulous.

Fontanelles, remaining open too long.

Fractured bones, to promote union.

Glands (lymphatics), enlarged, chronic.

Gonorrhea, with anemia.

Gout, rheumatic.

Hemorrhoids, chronic, in anemic or weak patients.

Headache, the head feeling and being cold to the touch.

Hernia, in anemic patients.

Housemaid's knee (swelling of the knee), with anemia.

Hydrocele (clear fluid in a cavity), if Nat Mur fails.

Hydrocephalus, water on the brain.

Inflammation of the eyes, during dentition, after Ferrum Phos.

Intestinal worms, predisposition to, in anemic patients.

Intermittent fever, chronic, in children.

Kidney disease (Bright's).

Lameness, rheumatic, obstinate, after Kali Mur.

Leucorrhea (discharge from the vagina), as a constitutional tonic.

Lumbago, if Ferrum Phos fails.

Lupus, if a partial manifestation of scrofulosis; see also Kali Mur.

Ozena (foul-smelling nasal discharge), with scrofulous symptoms.

Pains (rheumatic), in the head, worse during the night.

Pains in the head, worse with heat or cold.

Rheumatism, worse at night.

Rheumatism, aggravated by heat or cold.

Rheumatism, worse in bad weather.

Rheumatism, worse with change of weather.

Rheumatism, chronic, of the joints, with cold or numb feeling.

Rickets.

Skin affections, in anemic persons.

Suppuration (discharge of pus from infection), of bone.

Teeth, too rapid decay of.

Teething, disordered.

Teething, too late.

Teething, minor ailments caused by it.

Tonsils, chronic swelling,

Toothache, worse at night.

Toothache, worse in bad weather.

Tubercles (nodules), in the skin.

Whooping cough, obstinate cases.

"EVERY DISEASE WHICH AFFLICTS HUMANITY REVEALS A LACK OF ONE OR MORE OF THESE INORGANIC CELL-SALTS."

– J.B. CHAPMAN, M.D.

ASTROLOGY OF CALC PHOS
Capricorn: The Goat of the Zodiac
December 21 to January 19

Adapted from: *Cell Salts of Salvation* by Dr. George Carey

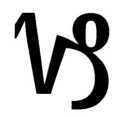 Persons born between the dates December 21 and January 19 come under the influence of the Sun in Capricorn, the Goat. Capricorn represents the great business interests – trusts and syndicates. Here many laborers are employed. Thus Capricorn symbolizes the foundation and framework of society – the commonwealth of human interests.

The bones of the human organism represent the foundation stones and framework of the soul's temple. Bone tissue is composed principally of the phosphate of lime, known as calcarea phosphate, or calcium phosphate. Without a proper amount of calcium, no bone can be formed, and bone is the foundation of the body.

A building must first have a foundation before the structure can be reared. Thus we see why the "Great Work" commences in the Goat. Lime is white – hence the "White Stone." In the book of Revelations (2:17) we read: "To him that overcometh will I give to eat of the hidden manna and will give him a White Stone, and in the Stone a new name written which no man knoweth saving he that receiveth it."

In the mountains of India, it is said, a tribe dwells, the priests of which claim that man's complete history from birth to death is recorded in his bones. These people say the bones are secret archives hence do not decay quickly as does flesh and blood.

Capricorn people possess a deep interior nature in which they often dwell in the "Solitude of the Soul." They scheme and plan and build air castles and really enjoy their ideal world. If they are sometimes talkative, their language seldom gives any hint of the wonderlands of their imagination. To that enchanted garden, the sign, "No Thoroughfare," forever blocks the way.

The governing planet of this earth sign is Saturn. The gems associated with Capricorn are white onyx and moonstone, and the colors are garnet, brown, silver-gray, and black.

In Bible alchemy (an esoteric interpretation of the Bible), Capricorn is represented by Judah, the fourth son of Jacob, whose name means "the praise of the Lord." John is the New Testament disciple associated with this sign.

CHAPTER 5

Calc Sulph

T issue is composed of living cells. By giving a tissue builder the deficient mineral salt in such a dose, fineness, and amount as can be assimilated by the growing cells, the most wonderful and speedy restoration to healthy functions is brought about in every case of curable disease. We know that these minerals are infinitesimally subdivided in the different kinds of food we take, thus rendering them capable of being assimilated by the cells. The cells of each tissue group receive their own special and peculiar cell salt.*

Calc Sulph (also known as calcium sulphate or lime sulphate) is one of the key components, along with Kali Mur, in the production of fibrin, the protein which supports skin tissue and blood-clotting. Lime (calcium) sulphate furnishes the cohesive, or plaster substance to sustain the integrity of tissue. The chief symptom of disease, indicating a deficiency in the lime salt, is suppuration, or discharge of pus, which is an exudation (discharge) formed by the breaking down, disintegration, and fermentation of epithelium. Calcium sulphate, by its union with protein, assists chloride of potassium (Kali Mur) to form epithelial tissue, or, at least, to hold it intact by its cohesive quality.

The third stage of catarrhs (mucus congestion), bronchitis, lung disease, boils, carbuncles (boils), ulcers, abscesses, or exudations from any part of the body indicates a lack of this tissue-builder. Calc Sulph not only sustains epithelial tissue, but, when administered in case of suppuration, it cleans out the heteroplasm (dissimilar tissue) from the interstices of tissue (between the cells) by causing the infiltrated parts to discharge contents readily, which prevents slow decay and injury to surrounding healthy cells.

The action of Calc Sulph is opposite to the work of Silica (Silicea), which hastens the process of suppuration in a natural manner, while the lime closes up a process that has continued too long. Thus are we made to

*This complete introductory section is adapted from:
The Chemistry and Wonders of the Human Body by Dr. George Carey.

realize the marvelous intelligence manifested in life's procession in the organism of man.

Chemical affinity is but a synonym of Infinite Intelligence in operation in the functions of man.

MATERIA MEDICA OF CALC SULPH

Adapted from: *The Biochemic System of Medicine, Materia Medica* by Dr. George Carey

Calc Sulph is used to clean out an accumulation of heteroplasm (dissimilar tissue) in the interstices of tissue (between the cells) to cause the infiltrated parts to discharge their contents readily and to throw off decaying organic matter so it may not lay dormant or slowly decay and thus injure the surrounding tissue. A lack of this salt allows suppuration (discharge of pus from infection) to continue too long. It controls suppuration. A decay of epithelial (skin or membrane) cells, after the infiltrated parts have discharged their contents, indicates a lack of this salt. This cell salt is needed in the third stage of all catarrhs (mucus congestion), lung troubles, boils, carbuncles (boils), ulcers, or abscesses.

While Silicea hastens the process of suppuration in a normal manner, Calc Sulph closes up the processes at the proper time if it is present in the blood in proper quantity.

The reason why Calc Sulph prevents the process or so promptly closes it up is because a lack of this vitalizer or inorganic worker in organic matter otherwise allows the epithelial cells to break down, allowing tissue to disintegrate. Then the fluids from the blood take up the waste and carry it off through some natural or artificial orifice.

Other salts, of course, are of some importance in such condition, but in true suppurations Calc Sulph is always the chief remedy because there can be no true suppuration when this worker is present in proper quantity.

Exudations (discharges) of albuminous, fibrinous (fibrous protein), or watery matter may take place because of a lack of other salts, even when there is no lack of Calc Sulph.

Characteristic Indications

(Note: Remedies in parentheses provide therapeutic support to Calc Sulph.)

Head – Suppurations (discharge of pus from infection) of the head or scalp, **with yellow, purulent (pus-containing) discharges** or crusts. Discharges of a sanious (watery, blood-tinged, foul) nature. **At crusta lactea (cradle cap,** condition afflicting infants and little children that creates scaly crusts on the scalp) stage of resolution, after taking Kali Mur.

Eyes – Inflammation of the eyes, when pus is discharging, third stage of inflammation. Abscess of the cornea. Deep-seated ulcers in the eye (Silicea). Thick, yellow discharges from the eye. Pus in the eyes. Inflammation of the retina, third stage. Inflammation of the cornea or conjunctiva, with characteristic discharge.

Ears – Discharges from the ear are thick, yellow, sometimes mixed with blood (Silicea). Deafness, when accompanied by these conditions.

Nose – Colds in the head in third stage of resolution, when discharge is thick, yellow, purulent, and sometimes tinged with blood. Chronic catarrh of head, with purulent discharge from either the anterior or posterior nares (postnasal discharge) (Kali Sulph, Silicea).

Face – Mattery (pus-containing) pimples on face (alternate with Silicea). **At puberty, pimples on the face,** when matter forms. Tender **pimples under the beard, with purulent, bloody secretions.** Swellings and nodules on the face, to abort or control suppuration (Kali Mur).

Mouth – Diseases of the mouth, if accompanied with purulent secretions.

Teeth – Ulceration at the roots of the teeth, with swelled gums and cheeks, to abort or control the suppuration.

Tongue – Inflammation of the tongue, when suppurating (Silicea).

Throat – All ailments of the throat in third stage of inflammation, or when discharging mattery secretions. Sore throat, quinsy (inflammation of the tonsils), and tonsillitis, when suppurating, or before pus forms, to prevent its formation.

Abdomen and stool – Discharge of pus or blood and matter from the bowels. Pus-like, slimy discharges. Abscess of the liver, with purulent discharge. Soreness in region of liver. Diarrhea, dysentery, with characteristic evacuations. Ulceration of the bowels. Bowels discharging mattery substance, or much constipation in latter stages of consumption (tuberculosis).

Urinary organs – Chronic inflammation of the bladder, when passing sanious or bloody matter (Ferrum Phos, especially if blood is bright red; Kali Mur).

Male sexual organs – Suppurating abscess of the prostate gland. Bubo (swelling of lymph glands, especially in the groin), syphilis, or gonorrhea in the suppurative stage, with sanious, purulent discharge (Silicea). Ulceration of the glands, with characteristic discharges.

Female sexual organs – Leucorrhea (discharge from the vagina) with thick, yellow, bloody discharge (Silicea). Gonorrhea, with the previously mentioned characteristics.

Pregnancy – Inflammation of the breast, when suppuration has occurred and pus is discharging (Silicea) from the breast (Kali Mur).

Respiratory organs – Last stages of consumption, when the expectoration is purulent, mattery, and sometimes bloody. If patient expectorates into a container, the mucus spreads out (Silicea). Cough, with hectic fever (characterized by irritation and debility, occurring usually at the advanced stage of an exhausting disease, as in pulmonary consumption) and sanious, mattery sputa (spit). Third stage of croup, pneumonia, or bronchitis. Generally indicated to be taken after Kali Mur. Pus forming in cavity of lung or pleura (mucus membrane enveloping the lung).

Back and Extremities – Suppurations of the joints (Silicea). **All wounds, when in the discharging stage** (if offensive, Kali Phos). Hip-joint disease; Ferrum Phos in the first stage; have patient rest (Silicea). Ulceration of bones (Silicea, Calc Phos). In consumption, **burning of soles of feet**. Third stage of inflammation, when the suppuration is superficial; check the discharge on the bandage to see if the amount of discharge is decreasing. Carbuncles (boils) on the back, to control the suppuration (Kali Mur, Silicea).

Skin – Skin affections, with yellow scabs (Kali Mur). Pimples, when discharging pus. Pimples under the beard, with discharge of blood

---

Calc Sulph Summary

ORGAN AND TISSUE AFFINITIES
Bones, tissues, connective tissues, mucus membranes.

MODALITIES
Symptoms worse < dampness, drafts, stimulants, evening, sleep, menses. Symptoms better > open air, bathing, doubling over, uncovering.

DEFICIENCY SYMPTOMS
Boils, yellow pus, contact dermatitis, burning, itching, inflammation.

DISEASE CONDITIONS
Abscesses, boils, inflammation, acne, eczema, yellow discharges, tonsillitis, tumors, ulcers, blood stained discharges.

and pus. Mattery (thick) scabs forming on the heads of pimples. Crusta lactea (cradle cap), with yellow crusts or secretions. Skin festers easily (Silicea) in smallpox, when the pustules are discharging. Boils, to abort them or to control suppuration. Neglected wounds, cuts, etc., when discharging pus and when not healing readily. Burns and scalds (if Kali Mur is not sufficient), when suppurating. Apply locally with a cotton ball.

Tissues – In all cases of suppuration, when the discharge continues for more than 7 days and the sore is unhealthy. Take Calc Sulph after a course of Silicea. Thick, yellow, or sanious discharge from any organ of the body. Suppurations and ulcerations of the glands; also apply locally. Ulcers of lower limbs (i.e., leg ulcers), with characteristic discharges. Purulent discharges in gonorrhea, syphilis, bubo, leucorrhea, catarrh, consumption, etc.

Febrile conditions – Typhoid, typhus, diarrhea, dysentery, etc., with sanious, bloody discharges from the bowels. Hectic fever in consumption and other diseases.

Sleep – Sleepiness and lethargy, when accompanied with hectic fever.

Modalities – Worse from getting wet. A warm, dry atmosphere will greatly assist the action of the remedy.

FACIAL SIGNS OF CALC SULPH DEFICIENCIES

Overall gypsum-white appearance. There may also be the presence of boils or abscesses.

Cold-white tone. Also characterizing a Calc Sulph deficiency, this coloring can be seen over the entire face.

Age or liver spots.

Pores may be enlarged.

Dirty appearance. There may also be acne discharging yellow matter.

Most authors on the subject have not described Calc Sulph facial deficiencies, but they are important to note nonetheless.

THERAPEUTIC INDEX FOR CALC SULPH

Adapted from: *Therapeutic Index* (1890) by Dr. W. H. Schuessler

Boils, as a third remedy, to reduce and control suppuration (discharge of pus from infection).

Burns and scalds, which are suppurating, as second remedy.

Carbuncles, to control the formation of pus (Silicea).

Catarrh (mucus congestion), cold in the head, with thick yellow, lumpy, mattery (pus-containing) discharge.

Cornea, abscess of, deep-seated.

Croup, if Kali Mur is not sufficient.

Crusta lactea (cradle cap, condition afflicting infants and little children that creates scaly crusts on the scalp), if Kali Mur is not sufficient.

Cuts, with thick, yellow matter, to control suppuration.

Diarrhea, mattery, bloody.

Dropsy (swelling), post-scarlatinal (scarlet fever), in rare cases in which Nat Sulph is not sufficient.

Dysentery, if mattery, slimy stools.

Eyes, inflammation of, with thick, yellow matter.

Fever, intermittent, back of tongue covered as if with drying clay.

Furuncles (boils), when pus forms.

Glands, lymphatic, threatening suppuration and when discharging pus.

Gonorrhea, in suppurating stage.

Hip-joint disease, suppurating stage.

Injuries, infected cuts, wounds, bruises, if suppurating.

Mastitis (inflammation of the breast), to prevent matter forming.

Pustules, nodules, when suppurating.

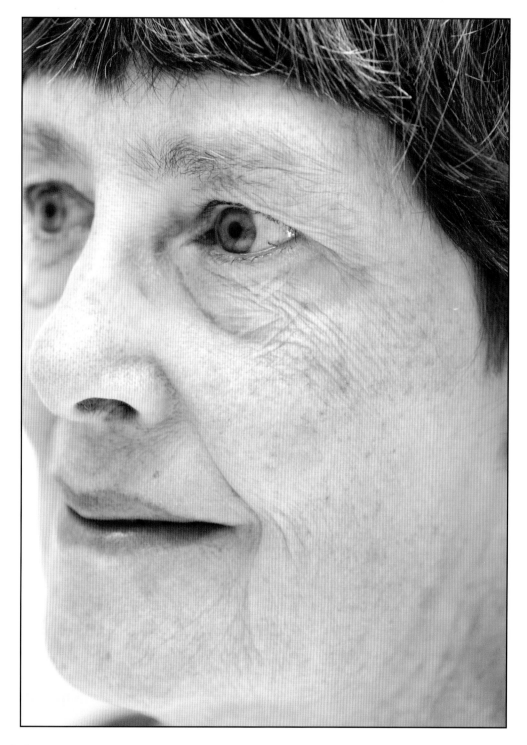

Calc Sulph (a)

This photo shows the Calc Sulph deficiency in the paleness of the chin area. This woman also has a Nat Sulph deficiency shown in the eye bags. Her wrinkles show a Silicea deficiency. The large pores on the tip of the nose are indicative of a Nat Mur deficiency. The shiny appearance on the nose is another sign of a Silicea deficiency.

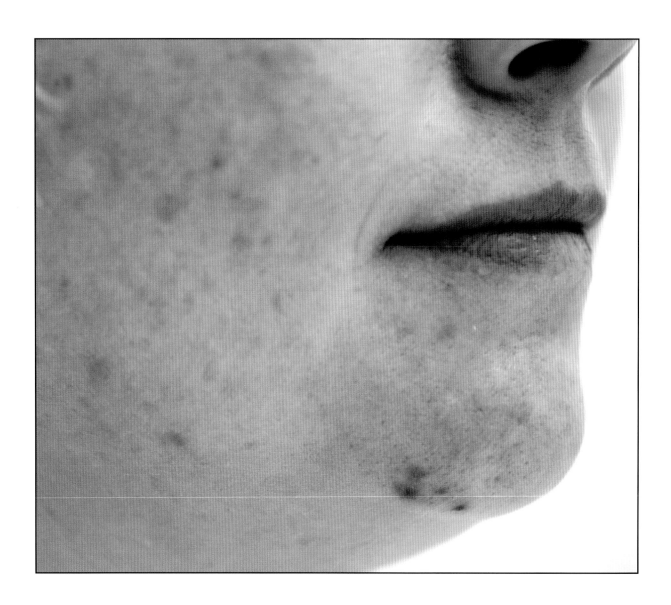

Calc Sulph (b)

The typically pale chin area, and with acne breakouts, indicate a Calc Sulph deficiency. This photo also shows a Nat Phos deficiency of a red chin, and a Kali Sulph deficiency due to the several brown spots and coloration. The chin area also has some large pores that indicate a Nat Mur deficiency.

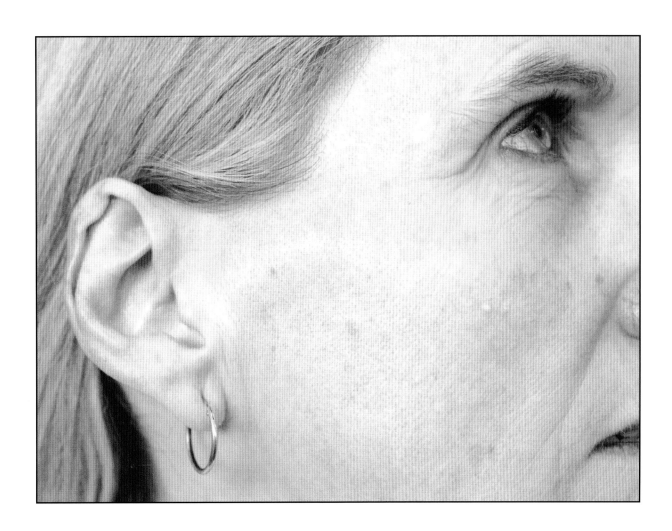

Calc Sulph (c)

Notice the pale white of a Calc Sulph deficiency around the lower cheek area. This subject also has a Mag Phos color overlay. The eyes have a greenish tinge of a Nat Sulph deficiency. The slight vertical lines parallel to the ear are a sign of a beginning Silicea deficiency.

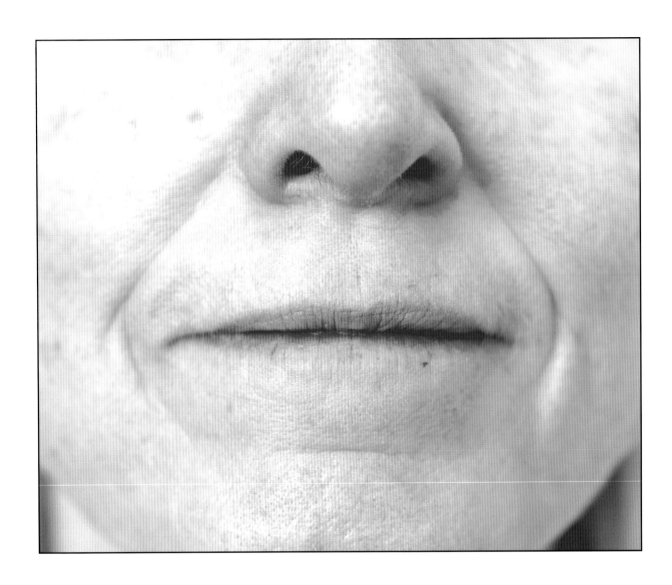

Calc Sulph (d)

This picture shows the face area with the pale Calc Sulph deficiency. She also shows a Nat Phos deficiency of the vertical lines above her upper lip. There are some large pores of the nose indicating a Nat Mur deficiency. The tip of the nose has the shine of a Silicea deficiency.

Scabs, forming on mattery heads of nodules and pimples.

Scarlet fever, sore throat, excessive swelling of soft palate.

Secretions, in inflammation, of bloody, lumpy matter.

Skin affections, with greenish, brownish, or yellowish scabs, if Kali Mur (the remedy to take at the stage when discharge was white) is not sufficient.

Suppuration, of articular joints.

Suppurations, having their seat in the connective tissue, arising from accumulations around the connective tissue channels.

Swelling, of the cheek, if Kali Mur is not sufficient and suppuration threatens.

Syphilis, chronic, third stage.

Throat, sore, threatening suppuration.

Tongue, coating at the back of, like drying clay.

Typhus, when diarrhea sets in.

Ulcers, also of lower limbs, if thick, yellow matter forms.

Whitlow (infected hangnails), when matter forms.

ASTROLOGY OF CALC SULPH
Scorpio: Influence of Sun on Vibration of Blood at Birth
October 24 to November 22

Adapted from: *Cell Salts of Salvation* by Dr. George Carey

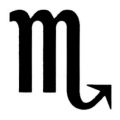 From Scorpion to "White Eagle" may seem a very long journey to one who has not learned the science of patience or realized that time is an illusion of the physical senses.

The zodiacal sign Scorpio is represented in human material organism by the sexual functions.

The esoteric meaning of sex is based in mathematics, the body being a mathematical fact. "Sex" in Sanskrit means "six." "Six days of Creation" simply means that all creation, or formation, from self-existing substance is by and through the operation of the sex principle – the only principle.

Three means male, father, the spirit of the male, and son. This trinity forms or constitutes one pole of Being, Energy, or Life – the positive pole. The negative pole, female trinity: female spirit, mother, and daughter. Thus two threes, or trinities, produce six, or sex, the operation of which is the cause of all manifestation. Those who understand fully realize the truth of the New Testament statement, "There is no other name under heaven whereby ye may be saved (materialized and sustained), except through Jesus Christ and Him Crucified." The possibilities of Scorpio people are boundless after they have passed through trials and tribulations, i.e., Crucifixion or "crossification."

One of the cell salts of the blood, calcarea sulphate, is the mineral ("stone") that especially corresponds to the Scorpio nature. Crude calcarea sulphate is gypsum, or sulphate of lime. While in crude form lime is of little value, but add water and thus transmute it by changing its chemical formation, and plaster of Paris is formed, a substance useful and ornamental. Every person born between October 24 and November 22 should well consider this wonderful alchemical operation of their esoteric stone and thus realize the possibilities in store for them on their journey to the "Eyrie of the White Eagle." Scorpio people are natural magnetic healers, especially after having passed through the waters of adversity, as the union of water and lime causes heat.

A break in the molecular chain of Scorpio salt, caused by a deficiency of that material in the blood, is the primal cause of all the so-called diseases of these people. These disturbances not only cause symptoms called disease in physical functions, but they also affect the astral fluids and gray matter of brain cells and thereby change the operation of mind into disharmony. Sin means "to lack or fall short," thus chemical deficiencies in life's chemistry cause sin.

The governing planet of this water sign is Mars. Mars is "a doer of things," also fiery at times, therefore, it is well that the Scorpio native take heed lest he sometimes "boil over." The gems associated with Scorpio are topaz and malachite, and the colors are golden brown and black. In Bible alchemy (an esoteric interpretation of the Bible), Scorpio is represented by Simeon, the second son of Jacob, whose name means "hears and obeys." Andrew ("to create or ascend") is the New Testament disciple associated with this sign.

CHAPTER 6

Ferrum Phos

One red blood corpuscle does not exceed the one hundred and twenty millionth of a cubic inch. There are more than three million such cells in one drop of blood, and these cells carry the iron to hungry cells in the most minute molecular form. Each one of the twelve inorganic salts has its own sphere of function and curative action. Thus we find Ferrum Phos (also known as the phosphate of iron, or ferrum phosphate) molecularly deficient in all fevers and inflammatory symptoms.*

Health depends on a proper amount of iron phosphate in the blood, for the molecules of this salt have chemical affinity for oxygen and carry it to all parts of the body. When oxygen carriers are deficient, circulation is increased to conduct a sufficient amount of oxygen to the extremities with the diminished quantity of iron, exactly as seven men must move faster to do the work of ten. This increased rate of blood motion is changed to heat, caused by friction, otherwise known as the "conservation of energy."

This heat, or increase in the temperature of blood, has been named fever, from the Latin word *fevre*, meaning "to boil out." The writer fails to see any relevancy between the word "fever" and a deficiency in iron phosphate molecules in the blood. From Hippocrates to Koch you will not find a true definition of fever outside of the biochemic theory. It is not simply the heat that causes distress in a fever patient, but it is the lack of oxygen in the blood due to a deficiency of iron, the carrier of oxygen.

A molecular break in the links of the chain of iron disturbs the continuity of other salts and thus causes more deficiencies. Chloride of potassium (Kali Mur) is usually the first salt called for after the disturbance in iron.

These mighty workers, iron and oxygen, cause all the blood in the body to pass through the heart every 3 minutes. The lungs contain about 1 gallon of air at their usual degree of inflation. We breathe, on an average, 1,200 breaths per hour; inhale 600 gallons of air per hour and 24,000 gal-

*This complete introductory section is adapted from:
The Chemistry and Wonders of the Human Body by Dr. George Carey.

lons daily; and iron and oxygen are the wizards that perform the miracle. When a deficiency in iron occurs, nature – chemical affinity – draws the blood inward from the surface of the body, in order to conserve this life-force so that the vital organs of heart, stomach, liver, lungs, and brain may continue to function. But the poor surface circulation allows the pores to close, and thus the waste matter that should escape by this route is turned upon the inner organs, causing exudations (discharges), catarrh (mucus congestion), pneumonia, pleurisy (inflammation of the membrane that envelops the lungs), etc. But these names are of no consequence. The lay student will clearly see that iron phosphate is indicated by certain symptoms in whatever part of the organism they may appear. Iron molecules give toughness and strength to the walls of veins and arteries and the minute blood vessels called capillaries and are, thus, the remedy for hemorrhages.

A child may touch a button that starts a complex machine, yet not understand the physics or the mechanism of the machine. So, many systems of healing may be the means of starting into action the workmen that may have become dormant. But when the workmen are deficient in the organism, and man's body is a chemical formula in operation, it would seem to be the sensible thing to do to furnish the needed chemicals.

There is but one law of chemical operation in vegetable or animal life. When a man understands and cooperates with that operation, he will call into being whatsoever he will; his organism will show forth the glory of omnipresent Spirit, and its "fearful and wonderful" mechanism will be the crowning glory of Earth.

MATERIA MEDICA FOR FERRUM PHOS

Adapted from: *The Biochemic System of Medicine, Materia Medica* by Dr. George Carey

Ferrum Phos colors the blood corpuscles red, carries oxygen to all parts of the body, and thus furnishes the vital force that sustains all of life. Without a proper balance of iron in the blood, health cannot be maintained. When a deficiency in this cell salt occurs, the circulation is increased, for the blood tries to carry enough oxygen to all the tissues of the body with the limited amount of iron at hand, and in order to do so must move rapidly; this situation is exactly as if seven men must move faster in order to accomplish as much work as could ten, moving at a slower pace.

This increased motion being changed to heat by the law of the conservation of energy is called fever. In no other medical writings will so simple and reasonable a definition of fever be found as the one offered by the biochemic pathology. It is not the fever or heat alone that causes the condition of unease in the patient, but the deficiencies in Ferrum Phos and a subsequent lack of oxygen. The interference with metabolism then caused soon prevents the functioning of other cell salts, with the result that they also lose their power of union with organic matter and are thrown out of the system. A deficiency in potassium chloride (Kali Mur) nearly always follows a deficiency in iron, unless the missing Ferrum Phos is quickly supplied.

A lack of Ferrum Phos, or a proper balance in the blood, is the cause of "colds." When a deficiency of iron occurs, nature, or the natural law, draws the blood away from the outer parts, the skin, in order to carry on the process of life more perfectly about the heart, lungs, liver, stomach, brain, etc. This, because of the closing of the pores of the skin, gives rise to accumulations of nonfunctional matters, which are thrown out by way of the mucus membranes, and forms the discharges of colds, catarrh (mucus congestion), pneumonia, pleurisy (inflammation of the membrane that envelops the lungs), etc. For all such conditions, whenever there is inflammation, under whatever name it may be known, Ferrum Phos is the chief remedy.

Without subjecting his patient to the delay necessary to diagnose the type of fever from which his patient is suffering, the biochemist gives Ferrum Phos because he sees in the symptoms a call for that tissue salt. Ferrum molecules toughen the cellular structure in the circular walls of the blood vessels, hence a lack of iron frequently causes a breaking down of the walls of minute blood vessels, producing hemorrhage. Ferrum Phos is indicated in hemorrhage from any orifice of the body. The alternating remedies are Nat Mur, Kali Phos, etc., according to the symptoms.

Characteristic Indications

(Note: Remedies in parentheses provide therapeutic support to Ferrum Phos.)

Mental symptoms – Rush of blood to the brain, causing delirium. Congestion of the brain from any cause. Maniacal moods. Hyperemia (accumulation of blood in any of the blood vessels). "Blood accumulated in any of the blood vessels causes want of proper balance of the iron molecules in the muscular fibers, which are circularly arranged around these vessels; thus relaxed, they lose their tonicity and do not support normal circulation" (Schuessler. Cerebritis (inflammation of the cerebrum), dizziness, wildness, madness, etc. (Calc Phos, Kali Phos). Delirium tremens (Nat Mur, chief remedy).

Head – Headache, with rush of blood to the head. Headache, when the pain is in the temples (Nat Phos); over the eye or on top of the head (Nat Sulph). Dull, heavy, bruising, throbbing, beating pains, generally accompanied by flushed face or fever. **Head sore to the touch**; pulling the hair causes pain; blind headache (causes partial or total temporary loss of sight). Vertigo; apply cold to relieve pains by momentarily contracting the excessively congested tissues; nosebleed also relieves vertigo by lessening the quantity of blood in the tissues. Headache with vomiting, when the matter vomited is undigested food (Nat Phos). Headaches, with red eyes. Inflammatory conditions of the scalp. Tic-douloureux (facial tics) (Calc Phos, Mag Phos).

Eyes – Acute inflammation of the eye (Kali Mur). **Inflammation of the eye in measles** and other eruptive diseases, with great intolerance of light. Acute pain in the eyes, more when moving them or attempting to use them. Dry inflammation, blood-shot, sometimes sore and watery (alternate with Nat Mur). First stages of retinitis. Abscess of the cornea, for the pain. **Granulation on the eyelids, feeling as if grains of sand were there** (alternate with Kali Mur).

Ears – Complaints of the ear, with inflammation. Earache, with beating, throbbing pain, due to catching cold. Sharp, stitching pains in the ear. Noises in the ear, roaring like running water, from a disequilibrium of the blood in the blood vessels. **Inflammation of the ear, first stage**, fever, and pain. Deafness from inflammation. Inflammation of the external ear, with **beefy redness** and burning. Tympanitis (inflammation of the inner ear).

Nose – First or inflammatory stage of cold in head. Taking cold easily (alternate with Calc Phos). Catarrhal fever. Chief remedy for bleeding from the nose, whether injured or not. Predisposition to bleed, in anemic, poorly nourished, or apoplectic subjects (Calc Phos, Kali Phos, Nat Sulph).

Face – Face flushed and burning, with headache, or when precursor to recurring headaches. **Flushed face with cold sensation in nape of neck.** Pale, pallid face, from a lack of red blood corpuscles in the blood (Calc Phos). Inflammatory neuralgia of the face. **Florid complexion**. Pains and heat in the face, when cold applications are soothing. Erysipelas (redness) of the face, for inflammation and pain (Nat Sulph).

Mouth – Inflammation of mouth. Stomatitis (cankers). Gums hot, swollen, and inflamed.

Teeth – Toothache, when due to an inflammatory condition. Inflamed gums or hot cheeks.

Toothache, when cold liquids are soothing. For feverishness in teething complaints, if Calc Phos is not sufficient. Pains are generally aggravated by hot liquids and by motion.

Tongue – Clean (coating-free), red tongue, showing an inflammatory condition. Tongue dark red and inflamed, with swelling (alternate with Kali Mur).

Throat – Throat sore, with inflammation. Throat dry, red, and inflamed. Ulcerated throat, with fever and pain. Tonsillitis. Quinsy, inflammation of the tonsils (Kali Mur, Calc Sulph). First stage of throat diseases, when there is pain, heat, or redness. This remedy reduces the inflammation; it should be alternated with Kali Mur, or if suppurating, Calc Sulph. Sore throat or loss of voice in singers and speakers, from overuse. First stage of diphtheria and all other throat affections (follow with Kali Mur and other indicated remedies).

Gastric symptoms – Inflammatory conditions of the stomach, pain after the smallest quantity of food. Burning, sore pain in pit of stomach. Region of stomach tender to the touch. Heartburn (Calc Phos, Nat Phos). Vomiting of undigested food or bright red blood. First stages of gastritis (Kali Mur). Persistent vomiting of food. Belching brings back taste of food. Cold drinks relieve pain. Apply heat (hot-water bottle, compress), which causes a counter irritation, thereby relieving the inflamed and engorged blood vessels of the stomach. Dyspepsia (poor digestion), with flushed face, and throbbing pain in the stomach. Vomiting of food, with sour fluids. "Stomachache from chill, with loose evacuation, caused by insufficient absorption from relaxed condition of villi" (Schuessler). Headache, with vomiting of food. Gastric fever (Kali Mur).

Abdomen and stool – First stage of all inflammatory conditions of the bowels. First stage of enteric fever, cholera, dysentery, peritonitis (inflammation of the membrane that lines the walls of the abdominal cavity), etc., when patient complains of feeling chilly. Constipation, when there is heat in the colon or rectum, causing a dryness of the mucus membrane. Diarrhea, caused from lack of absorption. Stools that are watery or that contain undigested material. Dysentery (Kali Mur, chief remedy). Bleeding hemorrhoids, with bright red blood, very painful (Calc Fluor); also apply in Vaseline locally. Worms, with indigestion and passing of undigested food (Nat Phos, chief remedy). Soreness and tenderness of the bowels, in acute cases (Kali Mur). Hepatitis. Hemorrhage of the bowels, when the blood is bright red and has tendency to coagulate quickly.

Urinary organs – Urinary incontinence from weakness of the sphincter muscle. First stage of inflammation of the bladder (cystitis), causing retention of urine, with pain and smarting when urinating. Burning after urinating (Nat Mur). Cystitis is often caused by retaining the urine too long, which should be avoided. Burning, sore pain over the kidneys. Urine dark yellow (Nat Phos). Bright's disease and diabetes, when there is feverishness, pain, or congestion in any part of the system, intercurrently. Suppression of urine because of being overheated, frequently in children; apply remedy externally over bladder. Wetting the bed from weakness of the muscles of the neck of the bladder (Kali Phos). If from worms (Nat Phos). Constant urge to urinate, if not chronic. Large quantity of urine (Nat Mur). Inflammation of the kidneys (nephritis).

Male sexual organs – Irritation and inflammation of the prostate gland (follow with Kali Mur). Varicocele (a varicose condition of veins of the spermatic cord, forming a soft tumor), bubo (swelling of the lymph glands, especially in the groin), orchitis (testicle inflammation), etc., first stage, when there is feverishness, pain, and throbbing. First stage of gonorrhea, for the inflammation; should be used in alternation with Kali Mur as a preventive when exposure to the disease has occurred.

Female sexual organs – Inflammation of the womb and vagina, to remove the fever, pain, and heat. Spasm of the vagina, with excessive dryness (Nat Mur). First stage of gonorrhea; apply remedy externally, placing a soaked cloth over the genital area. Metritis (inflammation of the uterus). Dysmenorrhea (painful menstruation), when there is congestion and fever, also vomiting of undigested food (Mag Phos). In the case of dysmenorrhea, Ferrum Phos should be taken between the periods as a preventive (Kali Phos). Menstrual discharge bright red.

Pregnancy – Morning sickness, with vomiting of food, sometimes with acid taste (Nat Phos). Inflammation of the breast, first stage. After-pains. If given immediately after giving birth, Ferrum Phos will heal any lacerations, thereby generally preventing the dangers of puerperal (postpartum) fever.

Respiratory organs – All inflammatory conditions of the respiratory tract in the first stage, for the fever, heat, and pain. Pneumonia, bronchitis, pleuritis, tracheitis (inflammation of the trachea), etc., in the inflammatory stage and, indeed, as long as the pain lasts (Kali Mur for the second stage or when the patient expectorates white mucus). **Hemorrhages** from the lungs, **blood bright red**. Expectoration scanty, streaked with blood. Soreness of the chest. Breathing short and hurried at the beginning or during the course of the disease, when there is heat and fever present. Cold in the chest, with hard, dry cough and soreness in the lungs (Kali Mur). Acute, painful, short, irritating cough. In the **beginning of all coughs and colds**, this is the first remedy. Croup and whooping cough, for febrile conditions. Asthma, for soreness of the chest. Painful hoarseness and huskiness in speakers and singers, when due to the irritation of the bronchi (Calc Phos). Congestion of the lungs, acute or chronic, with oppression and pain; breathlessness, pleurisy,

pain in the side, in the first stage. Local applications of hot water or mustard should be used when the pain is deep-seated, to produce counter irritation.

Circulatory organs – Inflammation of the blood vessels. Full, rapid, quick pulse in fevers. Palpitation of the heart, when due to inflammatory conditions. Carditis, pericarditis, endocarditis (all three conditions are inflammations of tissue of and around the heart), phlebitis, arteritis (inflammation of the artery), in the congestive stage. Anemia (Calc Phos). Chief remedy for aneurysm (Calc Fluor). Dilation of heart or blood vessels (alternate with Calc Fluor). Naevi (moles), varicose veins (Calc Fluor). Hyperemia (accumulation of blood in any of the blood vessels).

Back and extremities – Inflammatory pains in the back over kidneys and through the loins. Lumbago (Calc Phos). Stiff back, movement increases the pain. Rheumatism, for the inflammation and fever. Rheumatic fever. Stiffness of the muscles or neck from cold. First remedy in inflammation and infection, to relieve heat, pain, and congestion. Fingers painful or inflamed through rheumatism or other causes. Fractures of bones of the limbs, to meet the injuries sustained by the soft tissues, reduce inflammation, etc. In hip-joint disease, for fever, pain, and inflammation (Silicea). **Rheumatic lameness of the joints**, when fever is present (Kali Phos). Acute articular (joint-related) rheumatism, very painful. Rheumatism from catching cold. Pain is always aggravated by motion. Strains and sprains require this remedy in the first stage. In all cases, where practical, apply remedy locally.

Nervous symptoms – Congestive neuralgia after catching cold, with inflammatory conditions. Epilepsy, with rush of blood to the head and febrile conditions. Convulsions, with fever, in teething.

Skin – Inflammatory stage of all skin infections. Abscesses, carbuncles (boils), felon (infected hangnail), etc., require this remedy in the beginning to relieve heart pain and throbbing. Chickenpox, smallpox, erysipelas (redness of the skin from inflammation.), etc., in the initial stages, with febrile conditions (either alternate with or follow with Kali Mur).

Tissues – All injuries to the soft tissues, strains, sprains, cuts, blows, bruises, etc., call for this salt internally and externally. It will reduce fever, pain, and inflammation. In bone diseases or fractures, when the soft parts are inflamed and painful. **Anemia**; it makes the blood cells redder. In **dropsy** (swelling), when the disease is caused **from loss of blood** (alternate with Calc Phos). **In**

Ferrum Phos Summary

ORGAN AND TISSUE AFFINITIES
Lungs, ears (Eustachian tubes), blood, hemoglobin, nerves, circulation.

MODALITIES
Symptoms worse < motion; noise; nights and 4–6 a.m.; suppressed perspiration; on right side of body; consuming sour foods, cold drinks, meat, and coffee. Symptoms better > cold, bleeding, lying down, rising, passing stools, and solitude.

DEFICIENCY SYMPTOMS
Fatigue, low to moderate fevers, weak immune system, red face, nosebleeds, sore throats.

DISEASE CONDITIONS
Anemia, nosebleeds, sore throats, hemorrhages, low-to-moderate fevers, blood problems.

---

children and anemic individuals, bleeding from the nose (Calc Phos). **Hemorrhages** from any part of the **body, when blood is bright red and has a tendency to coagulate rapidly.** Hemorrhage from a small external vessel may be controlled by applying the remedy locally and binding on a compress tightly. In epistaxis (nosebleed), crush pellets of the remedy and snuff them up the nose. Plugging the nostrils with tissue or cotton is also sometimes necessary. In ulceration of the tissues, to control the fever and pain; use locally as well as internally in all cases where practical.

Febrile conditions – A feverish state at the commencement of any disease; continue to use as long as fever and inflammation exist, to control and subdue the heat, inflammation, and pain. This will, to a great extent, prevent the destruction of tissue. First stage of enteric, gastric, typhoid, typhus, rheumatic, and scarlet fever, measles, chickenpox, smallpox, etc., for the heat and congestion. Intermittent fever, with vomiting of food. Catarrhal fever, with quickened pulse and chilly sensations.

Sleep – Sleeplessness, from the weakened or relaxed condition of the muscular fibers of the walls of the blood vessels, allowing an accumulation of blood on the brain. If from worry or excitement, alternate with Kali Phos.

Modalities – Most of the ailments associated with a deficiency of this salt are congestive in nature and are therefore **relieved by cold and aggravated by motion.** Apply cold directly to the congested area, or relief will not be felt. If the inflammation is deep-seated, apply heat to relieve the engorgement of the deeper vessels.

FACIAL SIGNS OF FERRUM PHOS DEFICIENCY

Redness, in general, is a sign of a Ferrum Phos deficiency.

The acute redness of inflammation from a Ferrum Phos deficiency shows up as hot and feverish in the first stage. The patient will have **hot** burning cheeks and a hot forehead, as well as swollen, dry, red, and cracking lips.

Bluish-black circles under the eyes. I have seen cases in which the dark circles have completely disappeared in a matter of weeks after treatment.

Paleness of nose, earlobes, and lips reflects a chronic deficiency of Ferrum Phos.

A hung over or "didn't get enough sleep" appearance.

THERAPEUTIC INDEX FOR FERRUM PHOS

Adapted from: *Therapeutic Index* (1890) by Dr. W. H. Schuessler

Ailments, inflammatory stage.

Anemia, after Calc Phos.

Arthritis, rheumatic fever, at the onset.

Bright's disease, first stage.

Bronchitis, inflammatory first stage, before exudation (discharge) takes place.

Catarrh (mucus congestion), bronchial; the first remedy to be used in inflammatory stage.

Cholera, if inflammatory, first stage.

Cold in the head, first stage.

Colds, chills, first stage.

Constipation, from inertia of the lower bowel.

Convulsions, with fever, of teething children.

Cough, acute, painful.

Cough, acute, at the onset.

Cough, acute, from irritation of the windpipe.

Cough, acute, shaking, hard, with soreness.

Cough, acute, very painful, short, spasmodic.

Cough, acute, with feeling of soreness in lungs.

Croup, if it commences with violent fever.

Cystitis (inflammation of the bladder), first stage.

Delirium tremens, from alcohol withdrawal, also Kali Phos.

Diarrhea, from relaxed state of villi in intestines.

Diarrhea, stools containing undigested food.

Diphtheria, at the onset of the disease as the first remedy; shortens the healing process.

Dropsy (swelling), from loss of blood or fluids, second remedy.

Dysentery, if beginning, with much fever.

Dysmenorrhea (painful periods), with hot, flushed face and quick pulse.

Dyspepsia (poor digestion), with flushed, hot face; epigastrium (upper-middle region of the abdomen) tender to touch.

Earache, inflammatory (from cold).

Epilepsy, with blood rushing to the head.

Epistaxis (nosebleed), principally in children.

Erysipelatous (reddish skin) inflammations, with high fever.

Eyes, inflammation of, with acute pain, without secretions of mucus or pus.

Eyes, inflamed, with burning sensation.

Face ache, with flushing and heat.

Face ache, worse on moving; throbbing or pressing pain.

Feverishness.

Fractures, first remedy, supports the healing of the neighboring soft tissue.

Gastritis, inflammation of the stomach, with much pain; swelling tenderness in pit of stomach, especially if vomiting of food occurs.

Hemorrhage, if bright red, with tendency to coagulation.

Hemorrhoids, inflamed; apply remedy internally and externally.

Hemorrhoids, bleeding, blood red, tendency to form a gelatinous mass.

Headache, worse when stooping or moving; with vomiting of food.

Headaches, of children in general.

Hernia and prolapsus (falling down or slipping out of place of an organ or part), in otherwise strong individuals.

Hip-joint disease, first stage.

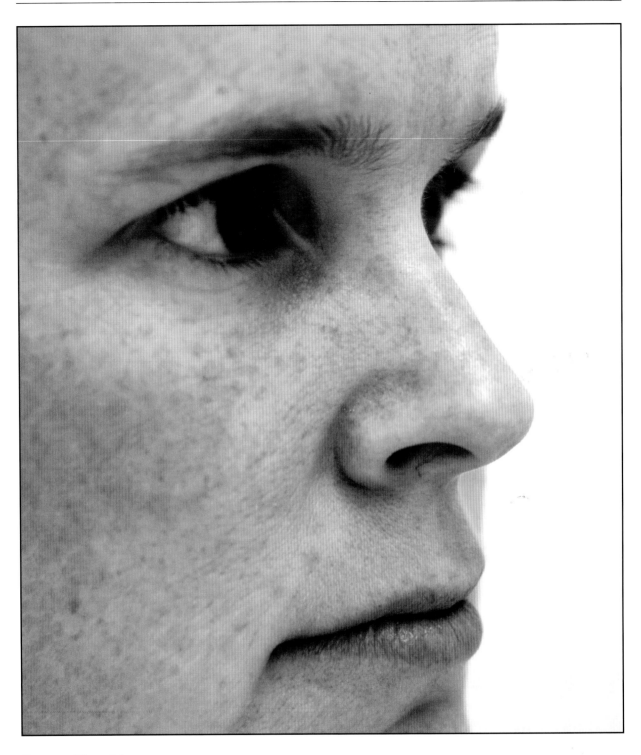

Ferrum Phos (a)

This woman has dark bluish-black circles of the eyes that start in the corner of the eye, showing the Ferrum Phos deficiency. She also has a Kali Sulph deficiency as seen in the brown spots. The eyes are deep set indicating a Silicea deficiency.

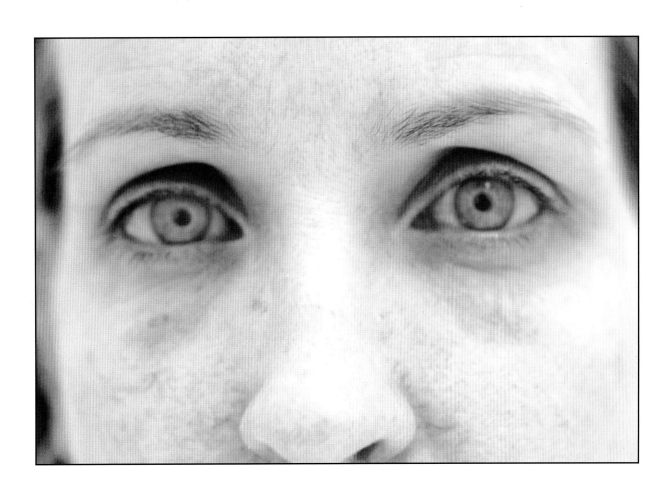

Ferrum Phos (b)

This person has dark circles under the eyes that show the Ferrum Phos deficiency. The face has a red Mag Phos deficiency overlay. The eyes are deep set and the nose is shiny, showing a Silicea deficiency.

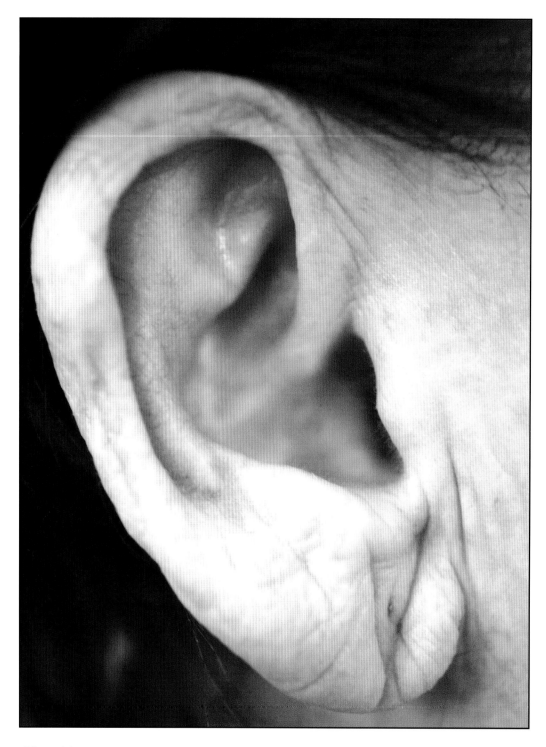

Ferrum Phos (c)

A Ferrum Phos deficiency is seen on the red ear-edges. The waxy appearance on the cartilage shows a Calc Phos deficiency. The vertical lines in front of the ear show a Silicea deficiency.

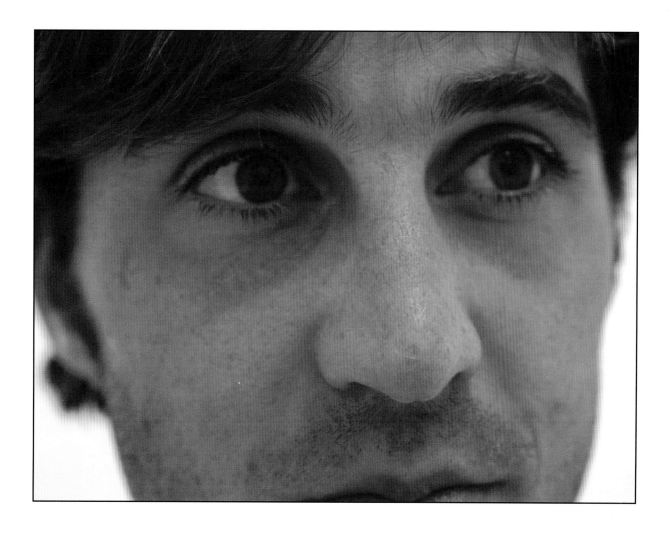

Ferrum Phos (d)

This man has strong dark circles under his eyes, showing a significant Ferrum Phos deficiency. He has the overall reddish coloring of a Mag Phos deficiency.

Hoarseness of singers or speakers, from overexertion of voice.

Incontinence (urinary), if from weakness of the sphincter.

Indigestion, from relaxed muscle fibers of the stomach.

Inflammation (hyperemia), in any part of the body.

Injuries, cuts, fresh wounds.

Intermittent fever, with vomiting of food.

Ischuria, suppression of urine, with heat; also in little children.

Lameness, recent rheumatic; also with feverish symptoms.

Lungs, inflammation of, first stage, until free perspiration is established.

Measles, in first stage, until other symptoms predominate.

Menstruation, with excessive red blood.

Morning sickness, with vomiting of food.

Ostitis (bone inflammation), with painful and inflamed neighboring soft tissue.

Palpitation, from changing conditions in the flow of blood to the heart.

Periostitis (inflammation of bone covering), with painful, inflamed soft tissue.

Peritonitis (inflammation of membrane that lines the abdominal cavity), first remedy, until profuse perspiration sets in.

Polyuria simplex (excessive secretion of urine).

Retinitis, in the first stage.

Rheumatism, pains felt only during motion or caused by motion.

Skin affections, in the first or inflammatory stage.

Sprains, use as soon as possible, externally and internally.

Stiff neck, if simply from a chill.

Stomachache, inflammatory, if pressure aggravates the pains.

Teething, with feverishness.

Throat, sore, dry, red, with much pain, inflamed.

Tinnitis aurium (sensation of noise in the ears), from flow of blood to the head.

Tongue, inflammation of, dark red, swelling.

Toothache, with hot cheek.

Toothache, worse with hot and better with cold liquids.

Uterus, inflammation of, first stage.

Vaginismus, mostly with heat.

Varicose veins, use both internally and externally.

Vertigo, from changing conditions in the flow of blood to the head.

Vomiting of red blood, with tendency to form a gelatinous mass.

Vomiting of undigested food.

Whooping cough, with vomiting of food.

ASTROLOGY OF FERRUM PHOS
Pisces: The Fish That Swim in the Pure Sea
February 19 to March 20

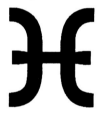

Adapted from: *Cell Salts of Salvation* by Dr. George Carey

Most everybody knows that Pikes (Pisces) means "fishes," but few there be who know the esoteric meaning of fish. "Fish" in Greek is "ichthus," which Greek scholars claim means "substance from the sea." The name Jesus is derived from the Greek for "fish"; Mary, "mare," means "water"; therefore we see how the Virgin Mary, pure sea, gives birth to Jesus, or fish. There are two things in the universe – Jesus and the Virgin Mary – spirit and substance. So much for the symbol or allegory.

From the Earth viewpoint we say that the Sun enters the zodiacal sign of Pisces on February 19 and remains until March 21. This position of the Sun at birth gives the native a kind, loving nature, making them sympathetic and kind to people in distress (Pisces natives often worry and fret when they cannot do more for their friends or those in trouble); they are also industrious, methodical, logical, and mathematical.

The phosphate of iron (Ferrum Phos) is one of the cell salts in human blood and tissue. This mineral has an affinity for oxygen, which is carried into the circulation and diffused throughout the organism by the chemical force of this inorganic salt. As the feet are the foundation of the body, iron is the foundation of the blood. Most diseases of Pisces people commence with symptoms indicating a deficiency of iron molecules in the blood; hence it is inferred that those born between the dates February 19 and March 21 use more iron than do those born under other signs. Iron is known as the magnetic mineral, due to the fact that it attracts oxygen. Pisces people possess great magnetic force in their hands and make the best magnetic healers.

The phosphate of iron (Ferrum Phos), in order to be made available as a remedy for the blood, must be triturated up to the third or sixth potency in order that the mucus membrane absorbents may take it up and carry it into the blood. Iron in the crude state, like the tincture, does not enter the circulation but passes off with the feces and often injures the intestinal mucus membrane.

The governing planet of this water sign is Jupiter. The gems associated with Pisces are chrysolite, pink-shell, and moonstone, and the colors are white, pink, emerald-green, and black. In Bible alchemy, Pisces is represented by Naphtali, the sixth son of Jacob, whose name means "wrestling of God." Philip is the New Testament disciple associated with this sign.

CHAPTER 7

Kali Mur

The cell salt Kali Mur (also known as potassium chloride or chloride of potash) is the mineral worker of the blood that forms fibrin (fibrous protein) and properly diffuses it through the tissues of the body.*

Kali Mur molecules are the principal agents used in the chemistry of life to build fibrin into the human organism. The skin that covers the face contains the lines and angles that define expression and thus differentiates one person from another. Fibrin is the building block for this and other connective tissue.

In venous blood, fibrin amounts to 3 in 1,000 parts. When the molecules of Kali Mur fall below the standard, the blood fibrin thickens, causing what is known as pleurisy pneumonia, catarrh (mucus congestion), diphtheria, etc. When the circulation fails to throw out the thickened fibrin via the glands or mucus membrane, this may stop the action of the heart. "Embolus" is the Latin word meaning "little lump or ball"; therefore, to die of embolus, or "heart failure," generally means that the heart's action was stopped by little lumps of fibrin clogging the auricles and ventricles of the heart. When the blood contains the proper amount of Kali Mur, fibrin is functional and the symptoms referred to above do not manifest.

Biochemistry has discovered the fact that the cause of embolus, diphtheria, fibroid tumors, and fibrinous exudations (discharges) are not the result of an oversupply of fibrin itself. These symptoms are due to a deficiency in the potash molecules that work with fibrin, to diffuse it throughout the organism and build it into tissue.

*This complete introductory section is adapted from:
The Chemistry and Wonders of the Human Body by Dr. George Carey.

MATERIA MEDICA FOR KALI MUR

Adapted from: *The Biochemic System of Medicine, Materia Medica* by Dr. George Carey

Potassium chloride (Kali Mur) should not be confounded with potassium chlorate or chlorate of potash, as it is an entirely different salt.

It is clearly shown by biochemistry that without the inorganic salt potassium chloride, no fibrin (fibrous protein) can be made; and it is further shown that the normal amount of fibrin cannot be held in proper solution in the blood without the proper balance of that cell salt. Fibrin results from the union of certain fibrin-plastic substances (proteins), but this union does not take place in the absence of the chloride of potash molecules. In venous blood, the fibrin amounts to 3 in 1,000 parts. Arterial blood contains less and lymph a still smaller amount. In inflammatory exudations (discharges) we find fibrin in the serous cavities – such as pleura (mucus membrane lining the lung) and peritoneum (membrane that lines the walls of the abdominal cavity) – and on the mucus membrane, as croup, diphtheria, catarrh (mucus congestion), etc. In all inflammatory conditions Ferrum Phos should be given in alteration with Kali Mur, for iron molecules carry oxygen, which becomes deficient when the proper balance is disturbed by the outflow of fibrin. It is quite clear that fibrin is created, or produced, by the action of the chloride of potash with the assistance of oxygen on certain albuminoids.

The white or gray coating on the tongue, mucus lining, or tonsils, is the fibrin that has become nonfunctional because of a deficiency in potassium chloride and oxygen. We find the fibrinous exudations also in discharges or expectorations of a thick, white slime, or phlegm, from any of the mucus membranes, or in white, powdery scales on the skin. The same material causes the enlargement of all soft swellings. (Hard swellings or lumps may be caused by the calcium salts and pure protein or silica.) The reason why Kali Mur relieves the effect of burns is because the fibrin in the tissue first succumbs to the effects of heat, and the chloride of potash, by its union with protein substances, produces new fibrin and supplies the deficiency.

Characteristic Indications

(Note: Remedies in parentheses provide therapeutic support to Kali Mur.)

Head – Headaches, with a thick, white coating on the tongue; vomiting of white phlegm or hawking of thick white mucus. Sick headache arising from sluggish action of the liver due to lack of bile, frequently accompanied by constipation. Secondary remedy for meningitis.

Eyes – All eye affections, when discharging a thick, white mucus (alternate with Kali Sulph when the discharge is yellow-green). Sore eyes, with specks of matter on the lids, or yellow mattery (pus-containing) scabs (Kali Sulph). Superficial flat ulcer arising from a vesicle. Secondary remedy in inflammations of the eye, with characteristic exudation. Granulated eyelids (with raised bumps, feeling as if grains of sand were in the eyes) (alternate with Ferrum Phos). Retinitis (inflammation of retina), with discharges.

Ears – Earache with a swelling of the glands and gray- or white-furred tongue. Earache, with swelling of the tonsils and eustachian tubes (Ferrum Phos). **Catarrhal conditions of the inner ear** (Ferrum Phos). Deafness from swelling of the internal ear; cracking noises in the ear upon blowing the nose or swallowing. Deafness from swelling of the eustachian tubes or thickening of the drum of the ear. Dullness of hearing from throat affections or swelling of the middle ear. Granulations; moist, gray or thick, white discharges from ear. Glands around the ear swollen; **noises in the ear; snapping and cracking** from imbalance in the air in the eustachian tubes (Ferrum Phos).

Nose – Stuffy colds in the head, with thick, white discharge and gray- or white-coated tongue. Catarrh, with characteristic white phlegm, not transparent. Dry catarrh, with stuffy sensation. Crusts in the pharynx.

Face – Cheek swollen and painful (alternate with Ferrum Phos). Face ache from swelling of cheek or gums.

Mouth – Canker of the lips of mouth, rawness of the mouth, swollen glands or gums. White ulcers (cankers) in the mouths of little children; look for characteristic grayish-white, dry, slimy look to tongue, with much saliva (Nat Mur).

Teeth – Toothache, with swelling of the gums or cheek, to carry off the pus and to prevent the further production of albuminoid substance. Gumboil, before matter begins to form (alternate with Ferrum Phos). (Silicea)

Tongue – Coating of **tongue grayish-white, dry, or slimy**. In inflammation of the tongue, for the swelling (Ferrum Phos).

Throat – Ulcerated sore throat, with white or grayish patches, white or gray tongue. Inflammation of the tonsils, with swelling and grayish-white patches. Quinsy (inflammation of the tonsils), acute or chronic; secondary remedy as soon as the swelling appears. For **diphtheria, this is the sole remedy in most cases** (can also alternate with Ferrum Phos). In diphtheria and all other throat diseases, gargle this remedy quite frequently (10–15 grains, 2x or 3x potency, in glass of water). Loss of voice. Mumps (alternate with Ferrum Phos; if there is much saliva or swelling of testicles, alternate with Nat Mur).

Gastric symptoms – Poor appetite, with gray- or white-coated tongue, indicating sluggish action of the liver. Dyspepsia (poor digestion), with white or gray-coated tongue, heavy pain under the right shoulder blade, eyes look large and protruding. Fatty, greasy food disagrees;

belching of gas, bringing back a greasy, sickening taste. Pastry or rich, fatty food causes burning and pain in the stomach. Indigestion, with vomiting of greasy, white, opaque mucus. Observe the white coating of the tongue. Take this remedy at once if gastritis, secondary stage, with white-coated tongue, or when caused by hot drinks (Ferrum Phos). Flatulence, with sluggishness of the liver. Stomachache, with vomiting of dark, clotted blood.

Abdomen and stool – Evacuations are pale yellow-, ocher- or clay-colored, denoting a deficiency of bile. Sluggish action of the liver, with pale yellow evacuations; pains in region of liver or under right shoulder blade. Sluggish action of the liver with **constipation**, white-furred tongue and protruding eyeballs. Jaundice, when caused by a chill, resulting in catarrh of the duodenum, white-coated tongue, light-colored stools, etc. Typhoid or enteric fever, white-coated tongue and abdomen with tenderness to the touch. Hemorrhage of dark, clotted blood. Constipation, in typhus fever. **Diarrhea with pale yellow-, clay-colored stools**; swelling of the abdomen, slimy stools. Diarrhea after eating fatty, greasy food. Dysentery, purging, with slimy sanious (watery and blood-tinged, foul) evacuations; pain in the abdomen, constant urge to pass stool; straining with great pain in the anus, causing patient to cry out. This remedy, alternated with Ferrum Phos generally cures painful, dysentery-like diarrhea (use Mag Phos for cramping pains). Constipation, light-colored stools, showing lack of bile, sluggish action of the liver, etc. Second stage of inflammatory diseases of the abdomen and bowels: peritonitis, typhlitis, perityphlitis, enteritis, etc. (Ferrum Phos is the primary remedy). **Hemorrhoids**, when the blood is dark and thick; alternate with other indicated remedies for the tumors, relaxed elastic fibers, etc.

Urinary organs – Cystitis (inflammation of the bladder), in the second stage, with swelling and discharge of thick, white, slimy mucus; also the principal remedy for the chronic form of this condition. Urine dark-colored; deposit of uric acid, when there is torpor and inactivity of the liver (Nat Sulph). Second stage of inflammation of the kidneys (Ferrum Phos is the primary remedy).

Male sexual organs – The principle remedy in gonorrhea. Inflammatory swelling of the testicle (orchitis) from suppressed gonorrhea (Calc Phos). Bubo (swelling of the lymph glands, especially in the groin), for the soft swelling. Chronic stage of syphilis, with characteristic white discharges, white or grayish tongue, soft chancres. Principal remedy; also apply locally.

Female sexual organs – Leucorrhea (discharge from the vagina) with characteristic milky-white, thick, nonirritating mucus. Ulcerations of the cervix uteri, with thick, white, bland discharge; apply remedy locally or use in a douche. Menstruation retarded or suppressed, too late or too early, when the discharge consists of dark-clotted, tough, black blood, excessive discharge. Neuritis, second stage. Congestion of the uterus, chronic or second stage, menstrual periods too frequent (Kali Phos). White-furred tongue; uterine atrophy, second stage, to reduce the swelling; if uterus is very hard (Calc Fluor).

Pregnancy – Morning sickness in pregnancy, with vomiting of white phlegm and white-coated tongue. Inflammation of the breasts (mastitis), secondary remedy, to control the swelling before pus has formed. Valuable remedy for puerperal (postpartum) fever in the early stages, with Ferrum Phos. For postpartum delirium, septic poison (infection), etc. (Kali Phos).

Respiratory organs – Second stage of all inflammatory conditions of the respiratory tract; the characteristic indication is a thick, tenacious, white phlegm or milky sputa (spit). Consumption (tuberculosis), with the above symptoms and heavy cough. Loud, noisy, stomach cough, with white expectoration, white-coated tongue, and protruding eyes. Short, spasmodic cough, like whooping cough (Ferrum Phos). Cough, with croup-like hoarseness. Principal remedy for croup for the expectoration (Ferrum Phos). Pneumonia, pleurisy (inflammation of the membrane that envelops the lungs), second stage, with thick, white, viscid expectoration. Asthma, from gastric derangement (digestive problem in which trapped gas applies pressure on the lungs), white tongue, mucus white and hard to cough up (for better breathing, Kali Phos). Loss of voice. Hoarseness from cold (Kali Sulph). Whooping cough, with characteristic expectoration, wheezing, rales, or rattling sound in the chest caused by air passing through thick, tenacious mucus in the bronchi, difficult expectoration.

Circulatory organs – Palpitation of the heart, in hypertrophic conditions, from excessive flow of blood to that organ. In second stage of pericarditis (inflammation of pericardium), to complete the cure (Ferrum Phos, chief remedy). Embolism (Ferrum Phos).

Back and extremities – **Rheumatism** of any part of the body, when there is white-coated tongue. Rheumatic pains, which are felt only during motion or increased by motion (Ferrum Phos). Chronic rheumatism, with swelling and pain from motion. Rheumatic fever, second stage, when exudation takes place, swelling around the joints. **Chronic swelling of the feet and legs.** Glands of the neck swollen. Hip-joint disease, for swelling before onset of pus formation. Ulcers on extremities, with characteristic fibrinous discharge (Calc Fluor). Bunions; use internally and externally (after Ferrum Phos). Chilblains (see Glossary) on hands or feet; also use externally for the itching (Kali Phos). Creaking of the muscles at the back of the wrist or arm on movement (after Ferrum Phos, if swelling remains). "This cell salt will remove the swelling by restoring the nonfunctional cells of the excretory and absorbing structures to normal action" (cited by Dr. Carey with no source given). All swellings are controlled by this remedy; if exceedingly hard, alternate with Calc Fluor.

Nervous symptoms – The specific or **chief remedy in epilepsy**, with white-coated tongue, protruding eyes, etc. (Mag Phos). Epilepsy, occurring with or after suppression of eczema or other eruptions. Wasting of the spinal cord (*tabes dorsalis*).

Skin – All skin diseases, when the eruptions are filled with white, fibrinous matter or when there are white, powdery scales on the skin. Skin diseases that arise from vaccinations. Eczema resulting from deranged or suppressed uterine functions. Eczema, with dry, white, powdery scales or albuminoid, whitish discharge, white-coated tongue; if very obstinate, alternate with Calc Phos. Eruptions, acne, pustules, pimples, etc, with thick, white contents. Erythema-redness (after Ferrum Phos). For swelling and white-coated tongue. Scruffy eruption on the heads and faces of little children (*crusta lactea*); alternate with Calc Phos. **The chief remedy** for vesicular, blistering **erysipelas** (redness); alternate with Ferrum Phos for the fever. Abscesses, boils, festers (small festering sores or ulcers), carbuncles (boils), etc., second stage, for the swelling before pus forms. Pimples on the face and neck, with thick contents. Herpes (shingles) (Nat Mur). Irritation of the skin, similar to chilblains. Chief remedy for lupus. Measles, hoarse cough, glandular swelling, white-furred tongue. After-effects of measles, diarrhea, white-colored stools, deafness from swelling of the throat, etc. Scarlet fever (alternate with Ferrum Phos). Sycosis (inflammation of the hair follicles), principal remedy.

Tissues – In anemia, this remedy should be used intercurrently, if skin affections present. Cuts and bruises (after Ferrum Phos, if there is swelling and exudation). Chief remedy for burns of all degrees; use internally and externally (moisten cloth or bandage with a strong Kali Mur solution and apply frequently). Fibrinous, thick, white, slimy exudations from any tissue after inflammation; if these exudations are not absorbed by the body, there is a swelling or

enlargement of the areas. **Chief remedy in glandular swellings**, proud flesh, exuberant granulations (both terms describe a fungus growth from a granulating surface that shows no tendency of scar formation). Enlargement of glands from scrofula (swelling of the lymph nodes). Sprains (after Ferrum Phos). **Chief remedy for scurvy**, with hard infiltrations (growths infiltrating into the tissue of the joints or hair follicles). Dropsy (swelling) arising from heart, liver, or kidney disease, or from obstruction of the bile ducts; generally creates a white coat on the tongue, whitish liquid (on aspiration). Dropsy of the extremities,

---

Kali Mur Summary

ORGAN AND TISSUE AFFINITIES
Fibrin (fibrous protein), glands, bronchials, mucus membranes, Eustachian tubes, ears, muscles, joints, shoulders.

MODALITIES
Symptoms worse < cold drinks; open air; drafts; night; dampness; sprains; motion; menses; fatty, rich foods.
Symptoms better > cold drinks, rubbing, letting hair down.

DEFICIENCY SYMPTOMS
Moderate fevers, white mucus conditions, allergies, varicose veins, glandular problems, chicken skin on the arms.

DISEASE CONDITIONS
Eustachian tube blockage, sinus problems, acne rosacea, varicose veins, white discharges, tonsillitis, fat digestion problems.

when the limbs have hard, shiny, glistening appearance; white mucus sediment in urine.

Febrile conditions – Second stage of inflammation or congestion of any organ. In gastric, typhoid, or enteric fever, second remedy, to restore the integrity of the affected tissue. Alternate with Ferrum Phos in scarlet fever, also as a preventive. Typhus fever, for the constipation. Puerperal (postpartum) fever, an important remedy in the early stage, with Ferrum Phos (Kali Phos). In rheumatic fever, for the exudation. Intermittent fever, with characteristic symptoms. All febrile conditions, with grayish-white, dry, slimy coating of the tongue.

Modalities – All stomach and bowel symptoms are **worse after eating fats, pastry, or any rich food.** Pains are increased and **aggravated by motion.**

FACIAL SIGNS OF KALI MUR DEFICIENCY

A milky appearance to the skin is one of the key signs of a Kali Mur deficiency. This appears on the skin under the eyebrows and around the eye sockets.

A milk moustache can appear over the upper lip, or it may extend to cover the entire cheek.

A milky-reddish coloring, 2-3 mm thick, may appear under the lower eyelid or on the upper eyelid.

A milky-bluish coloring, 2-3 mm thick, may appear on the upper eyelid.

There may also be a **milky-purplish coloring.**

Then it may appear as an **acne rosacea** (a rose-red coloration) with spider veins.

There may be a **chicken-skin appearance** on the upper arms or other areas. This is often seen as a Vitamin A deficiency.

THERAPEUTIC INDEX FOR KALI MUR

Adapted from: *Therapeutic Index* (1890) by Dr. W. H. Schuessler

Boils, to stop the swelling before matter forms; red swelling; use the Kali Mur as a lotion, but use no poultices.

Bright's disease (kidney inflammation), as a second remedy.

Bronchitis, second stage, when phlegm (mucus) forms.

Bruises with swelling, after the use of Ferrum Phos.

Cankers, thrush of little children, without great flow of saliva.

Catarrh, phlegm white, not transparent.

Chancre (syphilis swelling), principal remedy throughout, 3rd triturations, internally and externally.

Chapped hands or lips.

Cheek swollen; controls it well, reduces the swelling.

Cold, stuffy in the head, with whitish-gray tongue.

Cold, in the head, with white, non-transparent or yellowish-green discharge.

Cornea, superficial flat ulcer arising from a vesicle.

Cornea, opaque spots on.

Cornea, vesicle, blister on.

Cough, loud, noisy, stomach cough, with grayish-white tongue.

Cough with thick white phlegm, or yellowish green.

Cough, stomachy, noisy, with protruded appearance of eyes, or itching at anus.

Cough, croupy, hard, with white tongue.

Croup, the first principal remedy for the membranous exudation, unless fever is present. If so, Ferrum Phos for high fever.

Crusta lactea (condition afflicting infants and little children that creates scaly crusts on the scalp), principal remedy, to be followed by Calc Phos.

Cuts with swelling, as second remedy.

Cystitis, inflammation of the bladder, second stage.

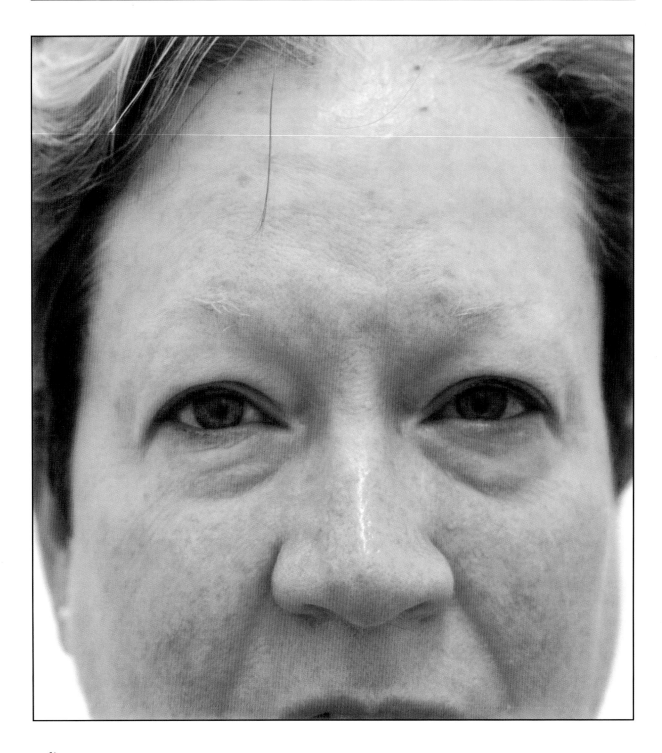

Kali Mur (a)

This photo clearly reveals the typical Kali Mur deficiency: notice the acne rosea-like cheeks and the nose with fine spider veins. She also shows a Nat Sulph deficiency of lower eye bags.

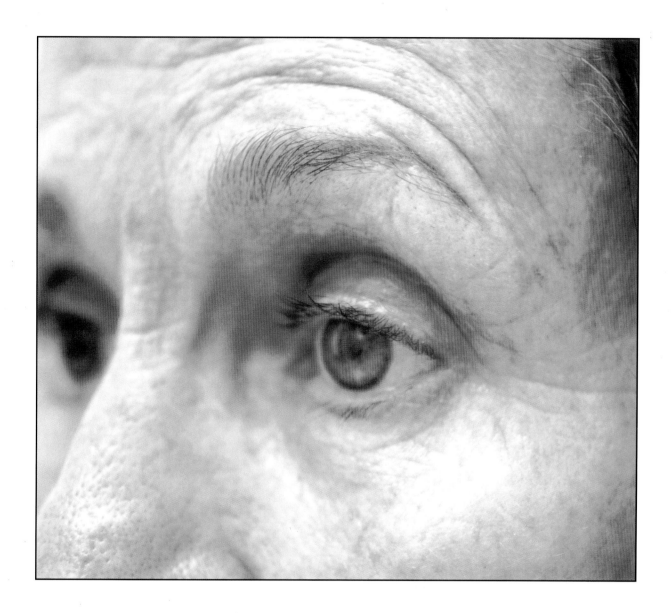

Kali Mur (b)

This woman has a milky coloration in her eyebrows, a sign of Kali Mur deficiency. She has a Kali Sulph deficiency shown by the brown spots. The deep-set eyes show a Silicea deficiency. The nose has large pores indicative of Nat Mur deficiency.

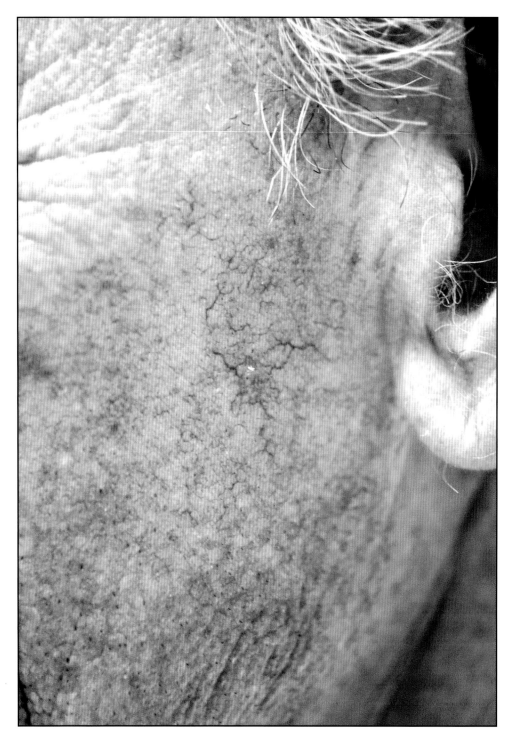

Kali Mur (c)

This cheek shows the Kali Mur redness with the more severe deficiency symptoms of spider veins. There is also a greenish overlay of a chronic Nat Sulph deficiency. This man has liver problems.

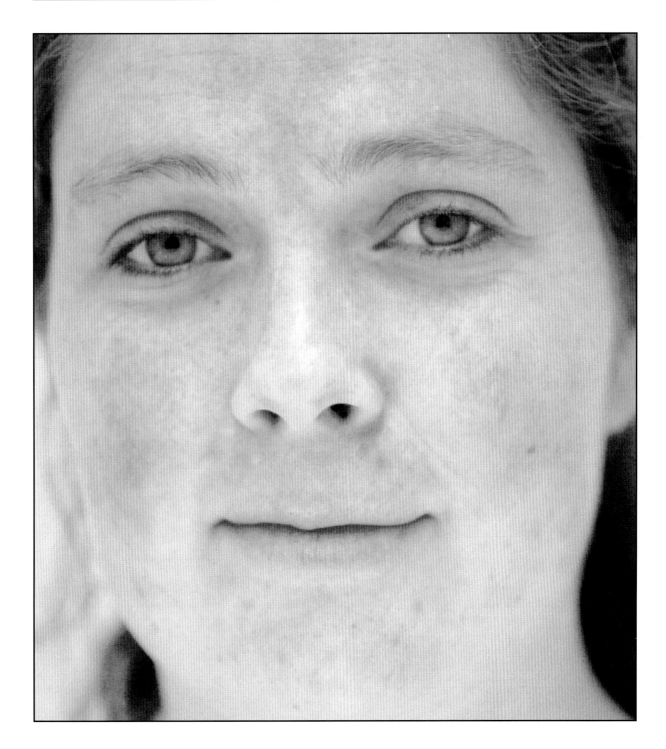

Kali Mur (d)

The hint of redness of the cheek indicates a Kali Mur deficiency. She also shows a Kali Sulph deficiency in the brown coloration. Here is another red overlay that shows a Mag Phos deficiency. The shiny nose indicates a Silicea deficiency.

Cystitis, chronic, the principal remedy.

Deafness from swelling in tympanic cavity (eardrum); primary remedy.

Deafness, from swelling and catarrh of the Eustachian tubes

Diarrhea, white slimy.

Diphtheria, the sole remedy in most cases after Ferrum Phos. Use gargle, 3rd triturations, 4-5 grains in tumbler of water very frequently.

Dropsy (edema) arising from heart, liver, or kidney disease.

Dysentery in most cases this remedy alone cures.

Eczema arising after vaccination with bad lymph.

Encephalitis, second stage, almost always suffices on its own.

Epilepsy if occurring with or after eczema.

Erysipelas, vesicular blistering (facial redness); the sole remedy.

Exudations (discharges), fibrinous in the interstitial connective tissues.

Eyes, sore on the lids, specks of matter, yellow mattery crusts; primary remedy.

Glandular swellings, first remedy.

Gonorrhea, principal remedy.

Gumboil, swelling, before matter forms.

Headache with vomiting, hawking up of milk-white mucus.

Hemorrhage, blood black, thick tough, clotted.

Hemorrhoids (bleeding piles), dark, thick blood.

Hip Joint disease, second stage, with red swelling.

Hoarseness, loss of voice from cold; in rare cases *see also* Kali Sulph.

Inflammation of the Lung, exudation, or second stage, after Ferrum Phos; this may cure without any other remedy; *see also* Calc Sulph and Kali Sulph.

Inflammation of Skin with subcutaneous swelling, or second stage or of soft palate, catarrhal, with white spots or patches.

Intermittent fever, white tongue, Nat Mur in special cases.

Lameness, rheumatic, and if with shiny red swelling.

Leucorrhea, (vaginal discharge) white, milky.

Lupus, principal remedy; see Calc Phos.

Mastitis (breast inflammation), second remedy, to control swelling.

Meningitis, as second remedy, will cut short the disease.

Menstruation, period excessive, dark, clotted, or tough, black like tar.

Menstruation, period lasting too long.

Menstruation suppressed.

Menstruation too frequent.

Mumps, this remedy will cure alone, unless there be great flow of saliva, in which case the choice will fall on Nat Mur. (Merc)

Morning sickness with vomiting of white phlegm.

Orchitis (testicular swelling), primary remedy if from suppressed Gonorrhea.

Palpitation from determination of blood to the heart; if Ferrum Phos fails.

Pericarditis (inflammation of peritoneum) as second remedy, following Ferrum Phos.

Pharyngitis (sore throat), with gray or whitish exudation, as second remedy.

Pleurisy (inflammation of the lining of the lungs), as a second remedy, after Ferrum Phos.

Proud flesh, requires generally this remedy only, internally and externally.

Rheumatic fever in the second stage; will, in most cases, suffice; red, shiny swelling.

Rheumatic pains that are only felt during motion, or increased by it; if Ferrum Phos does not remove it altogether.

Scales-white, floury, proceeding from blisters.

Scales on the scalp, white.

Scarlet fever, in mild cases it alone suffices.

Scurvy, hard infiltrations (from lack of vitamin C).

Small pox, the principal remedy; controls the formation of pustules.

Swellings in general are controlled by it.

Sycosis (skin eruptions), primary remedy.

Syphilis, chronic stage.

Throat, sore, ulcerated, with patches of white or grayish color; generally with the characteristic white tongue of this remedy.

Tonsillitis (Quinsy), chronic, with much swelling.

Toothache with swelling of the gums.

Ulcers with callous edges.

Uterus, congestion of.

Vomiting of blood, dark, clotted; or hawking of milky white phlegm.

"Whites" (vaginal discharge, leucorrhea), milky white mucus.

Worms, thread.

ASTROLOGY OF KALI MUR
The Chemistry of Gemini
May 20 to June 21

Adapted from: *Cell Salts of Salvation* by Dr. George Carey

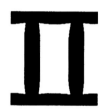 One of the chief characteristics of the Gemini native is expression. The cell salt Kali Mur/Kali Muriaticum (potassium chloride) is the mineral worker of blood that forms fibrin and properly diffuses it throughout the tissues of the body. This salt must not be confused with the chlorate of potash, a poison.

Kali Mur molecules are the principal agents used in the chemistry of life to build fibrin into the human organism. The skin that covers the face contains the lines and angles that define expression and thus differentiates one person from another; therefore Kali Mur, the maker of fibrin, has been designated as the birth salt of the Gemini native. Gemini means twins. Gemini is the sign that governs the United States.

Mercury is the governing planet of Gemini. The gems associated with Mercury are beryl, aquamarine and dark blue stones, and the astral colors are red, white and blue. While those who made our first flag and chose its colors personally knew nothing of astrology, yet the Cosmic Law worked its will to give America the "red, white and blue."

In Bible alchemy (an esoteric interpretation of the Bible), Gemini represents Issachar, the ninth son of Jacob, and means "price, reward, or recompense." In the symbolism and allegories of the New Testament, Gemini corresponds with the disciple Judas, which means service or necessity. The perverted ideas of an ignorant dark-age priesthood made "service and necessity" infamous by a literal rendering of the alchemical symbol, but during the present Aquarian age, the Judas symbol will be understood and the disciple of "service" will no longer have to submit to "third-degree" methods.

CHAPTER 8

Kali Phos

This salt is the great builder of the positive brain cells. Kali Phos (also called phosphate of potash, or potassium phosphate) unites with proteins and by some subtle alchemy transmutes it and forms gray brain matter. When the chemical possibilities of this brain builder are fully understood, insane asylums will go out of fashion. Nervous disorders of all kinds, sleeplessness, paresis, paralysis, irritability, despondency, pessimism, making mountains out of mole hills, crossing broken bridges that do not exist, and borrowing trouble and paying compound interest on the note – all these and many more abnormal conditions that make life a burden are caused by a break in the molecular chain of this nerve and brain builder.*

Man has been deficient in understanding, because his brain receiver did not vibrate to certain subtle influences; the dynamic cells in gray matter of nerves were not finely attuned and did not respond – hence, sin, or falling short of understanding. From the teachings of the chemistry of life we find that the basis of brain or nerve fluid is a certain mineral salt known as potassium phosphate, or Kali Phos. Kali Phos is the greatest healing agent known, because it is the chemical base of material expression and understanding.

Anything that prevents the formation of new cells as fast as old cells decay or die disturbs the equilibrium, and some pain or other symptom indicates that all is not right. This phenomenon is simply a telegraphic dispatch sent along the nerves to the brain to inform the ego, the "throne of understanding," that a deficiency exists – that the material necessary to keep up the processes of life is not sufficiently supplied at a certain place.

And why is it not supplied? Health is that condition of the system where a certain proper degree of heat is maintained, where there is a proper blending of positive and negative electrical influences, and where every tissue of

*This complete introductory section is adapted from:
The Chemistry and Wonders of the Human Body by Dr. George Carey.

the body is properly supplied with the right amount of blood, containing all of the elements requisite for building the new cells. This condition can be secured or maintained only by a proper amount of suitable physical exercise, a proper amount of food of the right kind, taken at reasonable intervals, and a judicious adaptation of the clothing to the temperature and occupation.

Anything which breaks up this balance injures just according to the degree of the adverse influence. In overeating, the alimentary canal (digestive tract) becomes clogged with undigested food. The nutrition, which should be set free to transmute through the walls of the intestines to be taken up by the absorbents and carried into the circulation, remains in the fiber of the food and passes out of the body and, of course, a deficiency at once exists in the blood.

Any disturbance in the molecular motion of these cell salts in living tissues constitutes disease. This disturbance can be rectified, and equilibrium re-established by administering a small dose of the same mineral salts in molecular form. *The Biochemic System of Medicine* is founded on physiology, anatomy, cellular pathology and chemistry as set forth by Schuessler and others in Europe, and many noted scientists of our own land.

Dr. Schuessler says, "My system or method of procedure is direct Biochemistry, because I use only tissue cell salts, substances which are homogeneous to those contained in the disease tissue. These salts, used properly, in a proper potency, cure all curable disease."

MATERIA MEDICA FOR KALI PHOS

Adapted from: *The Biochemic System of Medicine, Materia Medica* by Dr. George Carey

The gray matter of the brain is controlled entirely by the inorganic cell salt potassium phosphate. This salt unites with protein and by the addition of oxygen creates nerve fluid, or the gray matter of the brain. Of course, there is a trace of other salts and other organic matter in nerve tissue, but potassium phosphate is the chief factor, and has the power within itself to attract, by its own law of affinity, all things needed to manufacture this vital tissue. Therefore, when nervous symptoms arise, due to the fact that the nerve tissue has been exhausted from any cause, the phosphate of potassium is the only true remedy, because nothing else can possibly supply the deficiency.

The ills arising from too rapidly consuming the gray matter of the brain cannot be overestimated, and if all who are inclined to nervous disorders would carry Kali Phos with them, in tablet form, a large amount of sickness and suffering would be prevented. Kali Phos is one of the most wonderful curative agents ever discovered by man, and the blessings it has already conferred on the race are many.

Let the overworked businessman take it and go home good-tempered. Let the weary wife, nerves unstrung from attending to sick children or entertaining company, take it and note how quickly the equilibrium will be restored, and calm and reason assert themselves.

We find this potassium salt largely predominates in nerve fluid, and that a deficiency produces well defined symptoms. The beginning and end of the matter is to supply the lacking principle, and in molecular form, exactly as nature furnishes it in vegetables, fruits and grain. To supply deficiencies – this is the only law of cure.

Characteristic Indications

(Note: The remedies in parentheses are support for Kali Phos.)

Mental symptoms – Kali Phos, the great nerve and brain remedy, is indicated, and is the chief remedy in all mental disorders, when arising from a want of nerve or brainpower. A deficiency of this salt is indicated by the following symptoms: brain-fatigue from overwork, depressed spirits, irritability, impatience, nervousness; crossness of children

– ill-temperament, fretfulness, crying and screaming; fear; poor memory (Calc Phos intercurrently). Screaming of children at night during sleep, sometimes from worms; note color of tongue. Anxiety, gloomy moods, fancies, nervous dread, forebodings, looks on the dark side of life. Dull, no energy. Fainting and tendency to fainting in nervous sensitive persons. Insanity and other mental disorders. Delirium tremens (Nat Mur) softening of the brain, mental illusions and aberrations, grasping at imaginary objects. Backward-ness, shyness, sensitiveness; delirium during the course of any febrile disease (Ferrum Phos, Nat Mur). Puerperal (postpartum) mania, hysteria, fits of laughing and crying, melancholia, overstrain of the mind from continual mental employment, business worry, etc. Rest and Kali Phos will keep thousands of such cases out of the insane asylum. Sighing, weariness and depression. Somnam-bulism (sleepwalking) in children requires a steady course of treatment with this remedy. Homesickness, haunted by visions of the past (post traumatic stress syndrome).

Head – Headaches in nervous subjects, sensitive to noise, irritable. Headache, with confusion, nervousness, loss of strength, inability for thought, weariness, yawning and stretching, prostrated feeling and hysteria. Neuralgic headache with humming in the ears; better under cheerful excitement, worse when alone; tearful moods. Pains and weight in back part of head with weariness and exhaustion (after Ferrum Phos). Headaches in students and those worn out with mental work and loss of sleep; gone sensation at stomach. Pains are generally relieved by gentle motion or cheerful excitement; concussion of the brain, asthenic conditions, dilated pupils, etc. Anemic conditions of the brain, causing nervousness, dizziness and swimming of the head, when from cerebral causes. Vertigo from exhaustion and weakness (Ferrum Phos). Sleeplessness, noises in the head on falling asleep. Water on the brain (intercurrently).

Eyes – Excited, staring appearance of the eyes, dilated pupils (Belladonna), during the course of any disease. Drooping of the eyelids from weakness of the muscles. Squinting after diphtheria, when it is not spasmodic, but a weakness of the muscles. Partial or total blindness from decay of the optic nerve.

Ears – Deafness from want of nervous perception; noises in the ears and head, with confusion. Deafness with exhaustion of the nervous system. Ulcerations of the ear, when the discharge is foul, ichorous, offensive, sanious (foul discharges) or mixed with blood. Dullness of hearing, with noise in the head.

Nose – Catarrh (mucus congestion), with fetid discharge, foul odor, when the disease is located in the mucous membrane (see also Silicea). Ozeana (bad nose breath), with foul odor (Silicea). Bleeding from the nose in delicate constitutions, when the blood is thin, blackish, not coagulating; predisposition to bleed (alternate with Ferrum Phos).

Face – Neuralgia of the face from exhaustion of the nervous system and poverty of the nerve fibers. Face discolored and sunken, with hollow eyes. Pale, sickly and sallow face.

Mouth – Cankers, gangrenous canker of the mouth (alternate with Kali Mur). Ulcers of the mouth (Stomatitis), with very fetid, offensive breath and bad taste in the mouth; note also color of tongue.

Teeth – Toothache in nervous emotional subjects (Mag Phos). Toothache after exhaustion, mental labor, or from loss of sleep, better with gentle motion. Gums bleed easily; predisposition of the gums to bleed, with a bright red seam or line. Chattering of the teeth of a purely nervous character – not from cold.

Tongue – Tongue coated, like stale, brownish, liquid mustard. Offensive breath. Tongue very dry in the morning; as if it would cling to the roof of the mouth. Inflammation of the tongue, with excessive dryness or great exhaustion (Nat Mur).

Throat – After-effects of diphtheria, weakness of sight, partial paralysis, etc. Gangrenous condition of the throat, in the early stages. Croup, in the last stages, for syncope (fainting), nervous prostration, pale or livid countenance, etc., in alterations with the chief remedy, Kali Mur. Speech slow and indistinct, frequently indicating approaching paralysis. Paralysis of the vocal cords. In all throat diseases where there exists mental or nervous prostration.

Gastric symptoms – Inflammation of the stomach, when it comes too late under treatment, with weakness, debility and nervous prostration. Stomachache from exhaustion or depression, caused by grief, mental strains, worry, etc.; excessive hunger, unnatural appetite, frequently seen after febrile diseases. Hungry feeling after eating food; eats heartily, but appetite is not satisfied. Nervous depression, or "gone sensation" in stomach. Flatulence, with distress about the heart, or on the left side of the stomach.

Abdomen and stool – Dysentery, when the stools consist of pure blood, abdomen swollen, patient becomes delirious, stools have a foul, putrid odor, dryness of the tongue, etc. Diarrhea, with putrid, foul evacuations, depression and exhaustion of the nerves. In all diseases where bowel troubles are present, especially in foul or inflammatory conditions, the use of the indicated remedy in hot water injections should be resorted to. Flatulence, with weary pain in left side and distress about the heart; cholera, when the stools are profuse and have the appearance of rice-water. Typhoid fever, for the bowel troubles, malignant conditions, putrid blood, depression, etc. Prolapsed rectum (alternate with Ferrum Phos and Calc Fluor).

Urinary organs – Frequent urination, with passing of much water, frequently scalding. Inability to retain urine, from nervous debility. Incontinence from partial paralysis of the sphincter. Enuresis (wetting the bed) of children (alternate with Ferrum Phos, chief remedy); if

from worms, Nat Phos. Passing of blood from urethra; cystitis, for weakness and prostration. In diabetes (intercurrently), for nervous weakness, voracious hunger, sleeplessness, etc. Bright's disease for the disturbance of the nerve centers (alternate Calc Phos, for albumen).

Male sexual organs – Phagedenic chancres; gonorrhea, when discharging blood. Spermatorrhea for the nervous symptoms arising from the excessive sexual excitement.

Female sexual organs – Irregular menstruation, too late or too scanty, in pale, irritable, nervous sensitive women. Too profuse discharge, deep red or blackish red; thin and not coagulating menses, with offensive odor. Colic at menstrual periods, in pale, lachrymose, nervous women (Mag Phos). Suppression of the menstrual flow (Amenorrhea), with depression, nervousness and general debility. Hysteria at the menstrual period, nervousness and excitableness; also a feeling as of a ball rising in the throat. Hysterical fits of crying. Leucorrhea, when the discharge is scalding or acrid (alternate Nat Mur).

Pregnancy – Miscarriage, threatened in weak subjects (probably Calc Fluor). Mastitis, if the pus discharging is brownish, dirty looking, with offensive odor; also external application of the same. Puerperal fever, for the mania and derangement of the mental faculties. Labor pains, if feeble and ineffectual; also spurious labor pains. Tedious labor, from constitutional weakness. It will greatly facilitate labor, if given steadily for one month previous to birth.

Respiratory organs – Hoarseness from overexertion of the voice, exhausted feeling and nervous depression. Whooping cough, with the above symptoms. Asthma, large doses and often repeated, for the labored breathing and depressed system. Bronchial asthma, with characteristic expectoration and brownish coating of the tongue. Loss of voice from paralysis of vocal cords. Hay fever, for depression of breathing (alternate with Nat Mur, for the water conditions).

Acute edema of the lungs, spasmodic cough, threatening suffocation (alternate with Nat Mur, for the watery, frothy expectoration). Last stage of croup, pale, livid countenance, extreme weakness; syncope (in alternation with Kali Mur, chief remedy). Shortness of breath from asthma, or with exhaustion or want of proper nerve power, worse with motion or exertion. Involuntary sighing; sighing or moaning during sleep.

Circulatory organs – Pulse sluggish and below normal standard from enfeebled nervous system. Intermittent, irregular pulse. Palpitation, with nervousness, anxiety, melancholia, sleeplessness and restlessness. Palpitation on ascending stairs, with shortness of breath, from a weakened condition or nervous excitement; poor circulation, fainting and dizziness, with uneasy feeling about the heart, from weak action. Fainting from fright, fatigue or weak heart action, pulse low and hardly perceptible. Intermittent action of the heart after violent emotion, grief or care.

Back and extremities – Idiopathic softening of the spinal cord, with gradual molecular deadening of the nervous centers. Paralysis or partial paralysis of the limbs, Rheumatic pains, lameness and stiffness, worse from violent exertion, but relieved by gentle motion. Pains during rest; a bruised and painful feeling in the part affected; gentle movement gradually relieves. Acute and chronic rheumatism, very painful; parts feel stiff, severe in the morning, after rest or when rising from a sitting position; worse from exertion or fatigue; relieved from gentle movement; neuralgic pains in the limbs, with feeling of numbness (Calc Phos). Chilblains on the hands, feet or ears require this remedy, internally and externally, for the tingling or itching pains.

Nervous symptoms – Paralysis of any part of the body and of all varieties, require Kali Phos, the chief remedy. Partial paralysis, hemiplegia, facial, etc. Sudden or creeping paralysis of the vocal cords, causing loss of voice. Paralysis in which the vital powers are reduced, and stools

have a putrid odor, fetid breath, bad taste, etc. Locomotor, facial or creeping paralysis. "Neuralgic pains, occurring in any organ, with depression, failure of strength, sensitiveness to noise and light; improved during pleasant excitement and gentle motion, but most felt when quiet or alone." Nervous affections; patient irritable, impatient, dwells upon grievances, despondent, cries easily, "makes mountains out of molehills," etc. Nervous sensitiveness, feels pain very keenly; better when the attention is occupied by pleasurable excitement. Nervousness, without any reasonable cause; patient sheds tears while narrating her symptoms. Hysteric attacks from sudden emotion, with feeling of a ball rising in the throat, nervous fidgety feeling. Spinal anemia from exhausting diseases. Infantile paralysis. Epilepsy, for the sunken countenance, coldness and palpitation after the fit (in alternation with Kali Mur, chief remedy). Sciatica. Dragging pain down back of thigh to knee, accompanied by stiffness, from any cause, which has lowered the standard of the nervous system.

Skin – Eczema, with nervous irritation and over sensitiveness accompanying it (intercurrently). Felon (hangnail) or any other skin disease when the matter discharging becomes fetid. Pemphigus malignus. Blisters and blebs over the body, with sanious, watery contents. Skin withered and wrinkled. Putrid conditions in smallpox, malignant pustules. Itching of the skin, with crawling sensation; gentle friction is agreeable, but excess causes soreness and chafing (Calc Phos). Greasy scales on the skin, with heavy odor, Itching of the inside of the hands and soles of the feet where the skin is thickest. Irritating secretions. Chilblains, for the itching and tingling pain (Kali Mur, chief remedy).

Tissues – Wasting diseases, when putrid conditions are present. Hemorrhages from any part of the body, when the blood is thin, dark, putrid and not coagulating. Anemic conditions with characteristic symptoms of this salt. General debility

Kali Phos Summary

ORGAN AND TISSUE AFFINITIES
Nerves, brain, skin, temples, spleen, mucus membranes.

MODALITIES
Symptoms worse < excitement, worry, fatigue, pain, cold dry air, mental or physical exertion, eating, and early morning, puberty, being alone, sitting. Symptoms better > menses onset, sleep, eating, warmth, rest, gentle motion,cloudy weather, company.

DEFICIENCY SYMPTOMS
Poor gum and dental health, nervousness, depression, anxiety.

DISEASE CONDITIONS
Neurasthenia, fatigue, anxiety, panic attacks, sciatica, bedwetting, tinnitus, bad breath, yellow discharges.

and exhaustion, lack of energy. Exudations serous, ichorous, foul, offensive, sanious, mixed with blood. Exudations from the mucous linings, which are corroding or chafing (Nat Mur). Gangrenous conditions, early stages of mortification, to heal the conditions which give rise to it. Cancer, offensive discharges; greatly ameliorates the pain. Scurvy, gangrenous conditions. Suppurations, with characteristic discharge of offensive pus. Rickets, with putrid stools. Atrophic conditions in old people; tissues dry, scaly, lack of vitality. Septic hemorrhages. Persons suffering from suppressed sexual instinct, or from excessive sexual indulgence. General debility and exhaustion.

Febrile conditions – All febrile (fever) diseases, with low, putrid, malignant symptoms; typhus, camp, nervous or brain fevers, with low muttering. Sleeplessness, stupor, delirium, etc., high temperature, pulse below normal, or rapid and scarcely perceptible (Nat Mur). Intermittent fever, fetid, profuse, debilitating perspiration. Typhoid and scarlet fever, for the putrid, malignant conditions. Excessive and exhausting perspiration or sweating while eating, with weakness at stomach.

Sleep – Walking in sleep (somnambulism). Hysterical yawning; yawning, stretching and weariness, arising from nervous causes, sometimes with feeling of emptiness of the stomach, although food is not needed. Sleeplessness from nervous causes, often after worry or excitement. Wakefulness from high blood pressure to the head, stimulates the gray nervous matter, the gray nervous matter, thereby causing contraction of the arteries and diminished flow of blood to the brain.

Modalities – Symptoms are gradually aggravated by noise, exertion, arising from a sitting position, etc. Pains worse by continued exercise and after rest; symptoms are generally ameliorated by gentle motion, eating, excitement or pleasant company; worse when alone.

FACIAL SIGNS OF KALI PHOS DEFICIENCY

Ash gray appearance is the same as cigarette ash smeared on a white paper. This is a subtle layer over their normal skin coloring. This is most often seen on the **chin**, and the greater the area, the greater the deficiency. This is also seen on the **temples**, as well as the **lower eyelids** and **outer corner of the eyes.**

Sunken temples are indicative of a Kali Phos deficiency. We see this affecting the tissues, and the skin has lost its elasticity and shape. We see this in the sunken temples. This is often seen in a "hollow eyes" appearance.

Frosted luster to the eyes. This often shows the energy of the person. There is no Kali Phos deficiency if the eyes are sparkling, fresh and have a wakeful appearance. Kali Phos is the mineral for a weak life force and can be seen in the eyes.

Bad breath. This comes from the digestive system with a Kali Phos deficiency. The victims are often not aware of the problem. Their "significant other" often recognizes this. This type of bad breath comes from the tissues of the body. One can reverse the situation in 2-4 weeks of intensive Kali Phos use.

Facial deficiencies. Signs of Kali Phos are seen with a slight grayish appearance where local reserves are tapped by emotional trauma or continual stress. This is the time to take 4-12 pellets a day to head off serious problems.

Severe deep deficiencies are described above, and be sure to see a doctor where there may be a progression to more serious diseases.

Kali Phos can be taken with all other therapies, medications, etc. Deep deficiencies require 20-40 pellets per day for 6-24 months with some emotional support or constitutional homeopathic treatment.

THERAPEUTIC INDEX OF KALI PHOS

Adapted: from *Therapeutic Index* (1890) by Dr. W. H. Schuessler

Anemia, bloodlessness, from continuous influences depressing the mind.

Asthma, in often-repeated doses of 6x.

Breath, offensive, fetid, tongue coated like brownish liquid mustard.

Bright's disease, with corresponding symptoms.

Cholera, second stage.

Collapse, with livid, bluish countenance.

Concussion of brain, after Ferrum Phos.

Croup, if treatment is delayed till last stage, with extreme weakness, pale or livid countenance.

Cystitis, inflammation of the bladder, in asthenic condition.

Depression of spirits, melancholy, madness.

Diarrhea, foul; also, if accompanying any other disease, with putrid evacuations.

Diphtheria, in the well-marked gangrenous condition.

Dysentery, with putrid, very offensive stools.

Ears, noises in the, from nervous causes.

Edema, pulmonary (swelling of the lungs), with livid countenance.

Epilepsy, with pallor, sunken, countenance, coldness and palpitation after the fit.

Epistaxis (nosebleeds), bleeding of the nose, predisposition to it.

Evacuations (diarrhea), putrid, very offensive smell.

Face-ache, neuralgia, with great exhaustion after the attack.

Face-ache, neuralgia of nerves, over sensitive, pale persons.

Fits, from fright, with pallid or livid countenance.

Gangrenous conditions.

Gastric inflammation, if it comes too late under treatment, with asthenic conditions.

Headache, nervous, sensitiveness to noise, irritability, confusion.

Hemorrhage, blood blackish or light red, thin, not coagulating; *see also* Nat Mur.

Hysteria may be benefited by it.

Intermittent fever, fetid perspirations, profuse, debilitating.

Labor pains, if feeble and ineffectual

Mastitis (breast inflammation), if the pus is brownish, dirty looking, with heavy odor.

Menstrual colic, in lachrymose, oversensitive, irritable, pale females.

Menstruation, too late, in pale, irritable, sensitive lachrymose females.

Menstruation, too scanty, in similar constitutions.

Menstruation, too profuse, and heavy odor, pale red, or blackish red, and not coagulating.

Pains, laming, which are better with gentle exercise, worse on first rising up, or through exertion.

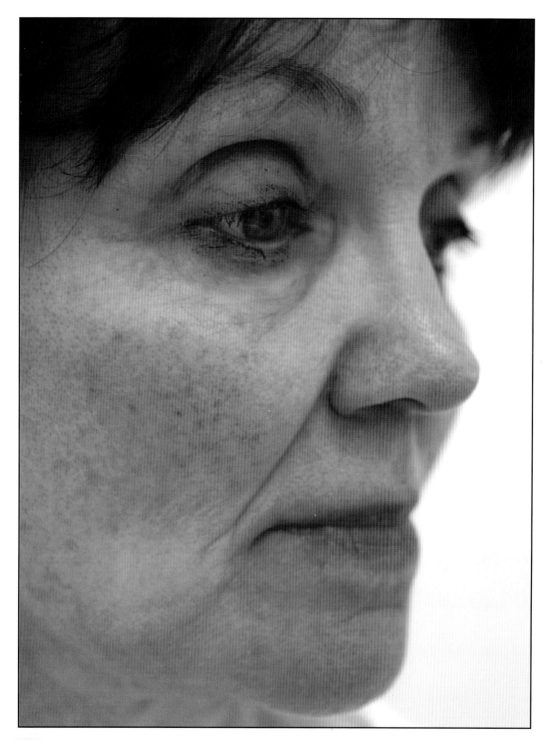

Kali Phos (a)

This woman has sunken temples and cheeks, and raised eyebrows. This is a severe Kali Phos deficiency, born out of a history of anxiety. The red cheeks are a sign of a Kali Mur deficiency. She also has a Ferrum Phos deficiency noted by the dark circles under the eyes. She has a reddened chin, which indicates a Nat Phos deficiency.

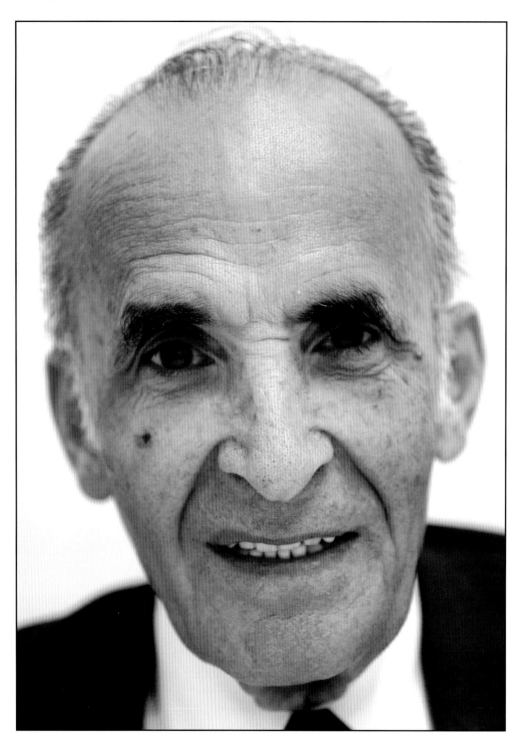

Kali Phos (b)

This man has sunken temples and cheeks, and the nervous-system symptom of the right-eye's raised eye-brow. These are signs of a nervous person with a severe Kali Phos deficiency. The waxy appearance is a Calc Phos deficiency. Large pores on the nose are indicative of a Nat Mur deficiency.

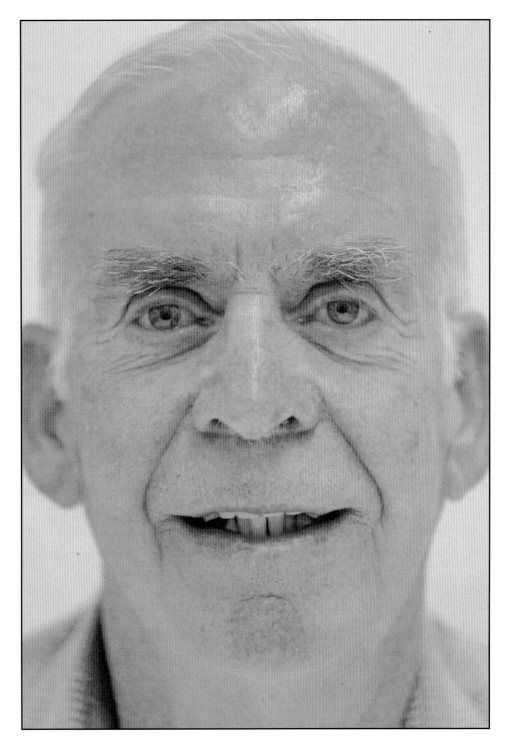

Kali Phos (c)

This man has slightly sunken cheeks and temples, showing a Kali Phos deficiency. The shiny forehead indicates a silicea deficiency. The red chin is a sign of a Nat Phos deficiency.

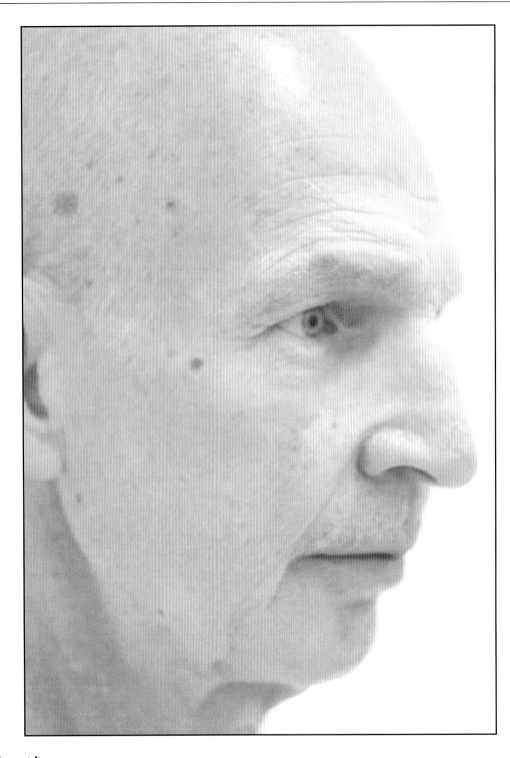

Kali Phos (d)

This person has metastasized cancer and has a yellow cast to his skin. There are also definite sunken temples. These outer signs point to a severe Kali Phos deficiency. The stress of cancer has caused the severe nerve deficiency of Kali Phos. There are also brown spots above the ear that indicate a Kali Sulph deficiency.

Palpitation, from nervous causes.

Purpura (purple coloring)

Rickets, atrophy, with putrid evacuations.

Scarlet fever, gangrenous condition, with typhoid symptoms.

Sciatica, pure neuralgic affection of the sciatic nerve in leg. (Possible spinal trouble.)

Septic bleedings (infectious bleedings)

Sleeplessness from nervous causes.

Smallpox, with putrid condition and exhaustion.

Stomatitis (ulcers of the mouth, i.e., cankers), with fetid offensive breath.

Suppurations, dirty foul matter, with offensive odor.

Tongue, coated like stale, brownish liquid mustard, offensive breath.

Toothache, of highly nervous, delicate, or pale, irritable persons.

Toothache, with easily bleeding gums.

Typhoid conditions, malignant.

Varicose veins, used internally and externally; *see also* Ferrum Phos.

Vertigo, from nervous causes, without gastric derangement.

Weakness of eyesight.

Weakness of sight if after diphtheria; *see also* Silicea.

Whooping cough; chief remedy.

ASTROLOGY OF KALI PHOS
Aries: The Lamb of God
March 21 to April 19

Adapted from *Cell Salts of Salvation* by Dr. George Carey

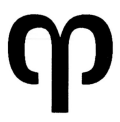

Astrologers have for many years waited for the coming discovery of a planet to rule the head or brain of man, symbolized in the "Grand Man" of the heavens by the celestial sign of the Zodiac, reigning from March 21 to April 19. This sign is known as Aries – the Ram or Lamb.

In ancient lore Aries was known as the "Lamb of Gad," or God, which represents the head or the brain. The brain controls and directs the body and mind of man. The brain itself, however, is a receiver operated upon by celestial influences or angles (angels), and must operate according to directing force or intelligence of its source of power.

From the teachings of the chemistry of life we find that the basis of the brain or nerve fluid is a certain mineral salt known as potassium phosphate, or Kali Phos. A deficiency in this brain constituent means "sin," or a falling short of judgment or proper comprehension. With the advent of the Aries Lord, ruler, or planet, cell salts are rapidly coming to the fore as the basis of material healing. Kali Phos is a great healing agent because it is the chemical base of material expression and understanding.

The cell salts of the human organism are now being prepared for use, while poisonous drugs are being discarded everywhere. Kali Phos is the special birth salt for those born between the dates of March 21 and April 19. These people are brain workers, earnest, executive and determined – thus do they rapidly use up the brain vitalizers.

In Bible alchemy, Aries represents Gad, the seventh son of Jacob, and means "armed and prepared" – thus it is said when in trouble or danger, "keep your head."

The Aries gems are amethyst and diamond, and the astral colors are white and rose pink. In the symbolism of the New Testament, Aries corresponds with the disciple Thomas. Aries people are natural doubters until they figure a thing out for themselves.

CHAPTER 9

Kali Sulph

The microscope reveals the fact that, when the body is in health, little jets of steam are constantly escaping from the seven million pores of the skin. The human body is a furnace and steam engine. The stomach and bowels burn food by chemical operation as truly as the furnace of a locomotive consumes by combustion. In the case of the locomotive, the burning of coal furnishes force, which vibrates water and causes an expansion (rate of motion) that we name steam.*

The average area of skin is estimated to be about 2,000 square inches. The atmospheric pressure, being 14 pounds to the square inch, a person of medium size is subject to a pressure of 28,000 pounds.

Each square inch of skin contains 3,500 sweat tubes or perspiratory pores (each of which may be likened to a little drain tile) one-fourth of an inch in length, an aggregate length of the entire surface of the body of 201,166 feet, or a tile for draining the body nearly 40 miles in length.

Let me repeat, for it is very important, the stomach is the furnace of man's body, and by the process of digestion, burns up food and furnishes the force to run the human engine, and thus enable it to inhale air, the material for blood, as water is the material for steam. In the manufacture of blood, through the complex operation of air passing through lung cells, arteries, etc., a certain amount of water is changed to steam, a portion of which escape through the safety valves provided by Divine Intelligence for that purpose. Sometimes the pores become clogged, and prevent the steam from escaping; then the vibration of the body changes and the person is sick. In many cases a disturbance in oil is the cause of the trouble. Kali Sulph (also known as sulphate of potash, or potassium sulphate) has an affinity for oil; it is the maker and distributor of oil. When this salt falls below the standard in quantity in the human organism, oil becomes non-functional – too thick, and thus clogs the pores.

*This complete introductory section is adapted from:
The Chemistry and Wonders of the Human Body by Dr. George Carey.

And does it not seem strange that medical science, which boasts of such great progress, can invent no better term than "bad color" for these chemical results?

Kali Sulph is found in considerable quantities in scalp and hair. When this salt falls below the standard, dandruff or eruptions – secreting yellowish, thin, oily matter, or falling out of hair – is the result.

Kali Sulph is a wonderful salt, and its operation in the divine laboratory of man's body, where it manufactures oil, is the miracle of the chemistry of life. Oil is made by the union of the sulphate of potassium (Kali Sulph) with albuminoids (proteins) and aerial (gas) elements. A deficiency of Kali Sulph in the molecules is the cause of oily, slimy, yellowish discharges from any orifice of the body, or from any glandular swellings, abscesses, cancers, etc.

MATERIA MEDICA FOR KALI SULPH

Adapted from: *The Biochemic System of Medicine, Materia Medica* by Dr. George Carey

The general field of action of this salt is the epidermis and the epithelium. In inorganic nature, sulphates and iron serve for the transfer of oxygen. When, in the surface layer of the Earth, a sulphate and any oxide of iron come into contact with organic substances undergoing a decomposition, they surrender their oxygen and form sulphuret of iron. This may be again decomposed through the access of new oxygen, so that sulphuric acid and some oxide of iron will be formed, which under suitable conditions will again transfer oxygen (Schuessler). Thus is explained the modus operandi of Kali Sulph, as an oxygen carrier, in which function it cooperates with Kali Phos. The oxygen in the lungs is taken up by the iron in the blood and carried to every cell in the organism by the reciprocal action of Kali Sulph and Ferrum Phos.

A deficiency of Kali Sulph causing a lack of oxygen in the skin and epithelial cells will give rise to symptoms of chilliness, heaviness and weariness, palpitation of the heart, anxiety, sadness, headache, and pains in the limbs.

Kali Sulph is also applicable to ailments accompanied by profuse desquamation (destruction) of the skin, including the stage of desquamation following scarlet fever, measles, erysipelas (facial redness), etc. This is, of course, due to its action upon the skin cells.

Characteristic Indications

(Note: The remedies in parentheses are support for Kali Sulph.)

Head – Dandruff on the scalp (internally, and as a wash, Nat Mur). Falling out of hair. **Headaches, which are better in cool air and worse in evening or heated room;** this is the characteristic modality for this remedy. Rheumatic headaches, with evening aggravations. Eruptions on the head, with secretions of decidedly yellow, thin matter; note the color of tongue. Scaling of scalp, with sticky secretions.

Eyes – Discharge from the eyes or eyelids, of yellow-greenish, serous matter, or yellow, slimy secretions; sometimes water. Yellow crusts on the eyelids. Inflammation of the conjunctiva, with characteristic exudations. Cataract, with dimness of the crystalline lens (Nat Mur.).

Ears – Earache, with yellow, watery discharge. Sharp, cutting pains under the ears. Catarrh of the ear and throat involving the Eustachian tubes, with yellow, slimy discharge, causing deafness. The ear should also be carefully syringed with the remedy once a day. **Deafness from swelling of the internal ear,** with characteristic discharge and evening aggravation; **note color of tongue.** After inflammation of the ear, when the secretion is thin, bright yellowish or greenish.

Nose – Catarrhal conditions of the head and throat, acute or chronic, with discharges of slimy, yellow or watery greenish matter; worse in evening or in a heated room. In the commencement of colds (in alternation with Ferrum Phos, to produce free perspiration); give frequently, and a majority of colds can be "broken." Colds, with dry, harsh skin, to induce perspiration. Stuffy colds, with large collections of greenish matter (Silicea).

Face – **Neuralgia** of the face, intermittent, shifting pain, evening aggravation; **better in cool air**, worse in heated room. Cancer of the face and nose (Epithelioma).

Mouth – Epithelial cancer of the lip, with characteristic secretions. Dryness of the lower lip; skin peels off in large flakes.

Teeth – Toothache; worse in the evening and in a warm room, better in cool air.

Tongue – **Coating of tongue yellow and slimy**, sometimes **with whitish edge**. Insipid taste.

Gastric symptoms – Catarrh of the stomach, with yellow slimy tongue. Dyspepsia, with characteristic coating on tongue. Indigestion, with sensation of pressure and fullness at pit of stomach. Indigestion, with pain (Nat Mur, Kali Mur). Colic pains in stomach, with slimy, yellow coating of tongue, or when Mag Phos gives no relief. Dread of hot drinks. Thirstlessness. Gastric fever, with rise of temperature in the evening; **note tongue symptoms**. In gastric fever, when the skin is dry and hot (in alternation with Ferrum Phos, to assist perspiration).

Abdomen and stool – In all abdominal troubles, with characteristic tongue symptoms and color of discharges from the bowels. Diarrhea, with yellow, slimy, purulent matter. Pains of a colicky nature, caused by sudden changes from heat to cold; **note color of tongue**. Abdomen cold to the touch. Sulphurous odor of gas from the bowels. **Hemorrhoids** (in alternation with the chief remedy, Calc Fluor), **when the tongue has a slimy, yellow coating**, or the characteristic discharge from the tumors. "Pain in abdomen, just above the angle of the crest of the ileum, on a line toward the umbilicus, deep within, beside the right hip." Bloating of the abdomen. Typhoid, enteric or typhus fevers, with evening aggravation and rise of temperature.

Urinary organs – Cystitis, with characteristic discharge of yellow, slimy matter from the urethra; third stage of the inflammation.

Male sexual organs – Gonorrhea, slimy, yellow or greenish discharge. Evening aggravation of syphilis, gleet, when yellow and slimy.

Female sexual organs – Gonorrhea, with characteristic discharges. Menstruation too late and scanty, with fullness and weight in abdomen; **note color of tongue**. Leucorrhoea, vaginal discharge of yellow, slimy or greenish matter.

Respiratory organs – Inflammatory conditions of the respiratory tract, when the expectoration is decidedly yellow-greenish and slimy. Bronchitis and consumption, with the characteristic expectoration or rise of temperature in the evening; **note the color of the tongue**. Bronchial asthma, with yellow expectoration, for the labored breathing, Kali Phos. **Cough**, with the distinctly yellow sputa, which is **worse in the evening, or in a heated atmosphere; better in the cool, open air**. Cough when the expectoration is yellow, tenacious and ropy, causing it to slip back, and is generally swallowed. Croupy hoarseness (chief remedy, Kali Mur). Sensation of weariness in the pharynx; speaking is fatiguing. In **whooping cough, for yellow slimy expectoration**; for the whoop, Mag Phos. Pneumonia, with yellow phlegm, greatly rattling and gurgling of mucus in the chest, suffocative, smothering feeling in the heated room, must go in the open air for relief.

Circulatory organs – Pulse quick, with throbbing, boring pain over crest of ileum; pallid face. Temperature rises toward evening. Pulse very slow and sluggish, sometimes met with in low fevers, which have a tendency toward blood poisoning; **skin is hot, very dry and harsh.**

Back and extremities – Rheumatic pains in the joints, when they are disposed to wander. Rheumatism of any part of the body, when of a shifting or wandering nature, with other characteristic indications for this remedy. Neuralgic or rheumatic pains in the back, limbs or any part of the body, when worse in the evening or in a warm room; with amelioration in the cool, open air. Fungoid inflammation of joints.

Nervous symptoms – Pains of neuralgic nature, with tendency to shift, from one place to another.

Skin – All sores on the skin, when exuding a thin, yellow, watery matter, sometimes with dryness and desquamation of the surrounding skin. Skin scales freely on a sticky base. Skin is dry, hot and burning, lack of perspiration. Scarlet fever, measles, smallpox, etc., when the rash has been suppressed, "struck in," skin is dry and hot. **This salt also greatly aids desquamation in eruptive diseases, and assists in the formation of new skin.** Diseased conditions of the nails, interrupted in growth (chief remedy, Silicea). Dandruff; epithelial cancer, with characteristic discharge of thin, yellow, purulent matter; also local applications of the remedy. Eczema, when the symptoms of this remedy are present, also when the eruption is suddenly suppressed. In fevers, when the skin is dry and hot (to promote perspiration, should be given in alternation with Ferrum Phos).

Tissues – All inflammations, when there is watery, yellow or greenish, purulent secretions. Epithelial cancer, with characteristic discharges; serous, watery exudations from any membrane.

Febrile conditions – Fevers (gastric, typhoid, scarlet, enteric, etc.) when the **temperature rises in the evening.** In fevers, when blood poisoning threatens. It assists in promoting perspiration; it should, therefore, be given frequently in alternation with Ferrum Phos. In eruptive fevers, to aid desquamation.

Kali Sulph Summary

ORGAN AND TISSUE AFFINITIES
Respiratory, skin, glands, mucus membranes, pancreas, pigmentation.

MODALITIES
Symptoms worse < warm air, heated rooms, noise, evenings, consolation, after eating.
Symptoms better > walking, cool air, fasting, open air, heated room.

DEFICIENCY SYMPTOMS
Possible thyroid indications, high fevers, hyper- or hypo-pigmentation, freckles, liver or old-age spots. Brownness of skin coloring.

DISEASE CONDITIONS
High fevers, vitiligo (lack of pigmentation), freckles, eczema, sinusitis, psoriasis, asthma.

Note: This remedy is the chronic Pulsatilla. The symptoms such as wandering pains, changeable discharges, moodiness, etc. are the same.

Modalities – Aggravation in a heated room or in the evening. Always better in the cool, open air. Rise of temperature in the evening until midnight.

FACIAL SIGNS OF KALI SULPH DEFICIENCY

Brownish yellow appearance. This can be confused with Calc Fluor and its brownish black coloration.

The **A-form appearance** is a classic, brownish-yellow coloring on the root of the nose that extends out in a pyramid or "A" shape to the chin. You may also notice a "milk moustache" of Kali Mur in the midst of this. Note: one must also take into account a possible suntan and cultural color variations.

Pigmentation spots are seen as lacking, as in vitiligo, or as liver spots or a pregnancy mask appearance.

Freckles are abnormal in adults and must be seen as a Kali Sulf deficiency, and may indicate some sort of liver problem.

Age spots, although similar to the above situation, may also indicate a Calc Fluor deficiency. Both must be addressed. These can be anywhere on the body.

The pregnancy mask, a brown pigmentation can be seen especially around the neck and around the ears and cheeks, indicative of some sort of hormonal (negative) shift. Hormone replacement therapy or birth control pills may contribute. Heavy coffee consumption and smoking can also contribute because all of the above may cause Kali Sulf deficiencies.

THERAPEUTIC INDEX FOR KALI SULPH

Adapted from *Therapeutic Index* (1890) by Dr. W. H. Schuessler

Catarrhs, with yellow slimy secretions.
Dandruff, yellow scales on scalp.
Deafness, from swelling of tympanitic cavity (eardrum), if tongue or other accompanying symptoms point to it.
Deafness, throat, with catarrh and swelling of Eustachian tubes (also Kali Mur), with symptoms as above.
Ears, secretion of thin yellow slimy matter.
Face-ache, aggravated in the warm room and in the evening; improved in the cool, open air.
Headache, that grows worse in warm room and in evening, and is better in cool, open air.

Inflammations, with yellow, slimy secretions or excessive serous, if Kali Mur does not absorb these completely.
Lungs, inflammation of, if the loose, rattling yellow phlegm cannot be coughed up easily.
Menstruation, too late and too scanty.
Rheumatic fever, articular (joint), if Kali Mur does not quite suffice; third remedy.
Rheumatic wandering pains in the joints.
Scarlet fever, assists the desquamation, and meets most of the concurrent symptoms.
Skin, yellow, sticky secretions on limited portions.
Smallpox, assists the falling off of the crusts.
Tongue, yellow slimy coating.
Toothache, aggravated in the warm room and in the evening, but better in the cool, open air.

ASTROLOGY OF KALI SULPH
Virgo: The Virgin Mary
August 22 to September 23

Adapted from: *Cell Salts of Salvation* by Dr. George Carey

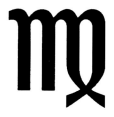

Virgin means pure. Mary, Marie, or Mare (Mar) means water. The letter M is simply the sign of Aquarius, The Water Bearer. Virgin Mary means pure sea, or water. Jesus is derived from a Greek word meaning "fish." Out of the pure sea, or water, come fish. Out of a woman's body comes the "word made flesh." All substance comes forth from air, which is a higher potency of water.

All substance is fish, or the substance of Jesus. This substance is made to say, "Eat, this is My body; drink, this is My blood." There is nothing from which flesh and blood can be made, but the one universal Air, Energy, or Spirit, in which man has his being. All tangible elements are the effects of certain rates of motion of the intangible

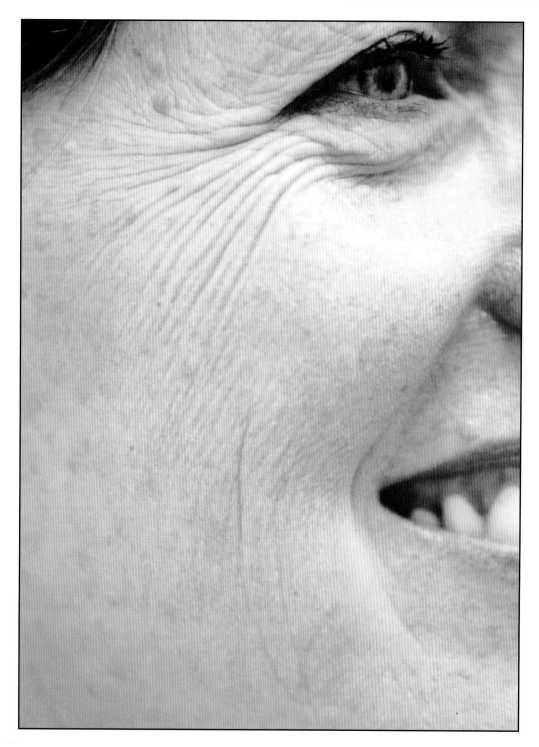

Kali Sulph (a)

This Kali Sulph deficiency is seen from the brown spots on the cheek. There is also a severe Calc Fluor deficiency seen on the outer edge of the eye with the developed crow's-feet. The lower eye-bag indicates a Nat Sulph deficiency.

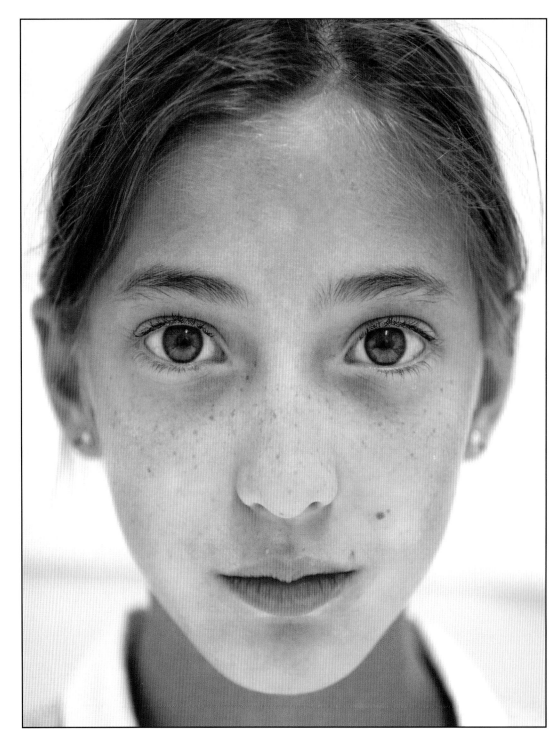

Kali Sulph (b)

This photo shows a severe Kali Sulph deficiency – both brown freckles and also white patches. Generally one would see either an excess or a lack of pigmentation with the Kali Sulph deficiency. This subject had both. One can also see a brownish-black circle under the eye, pointing to a Calc Fluor deficiency.

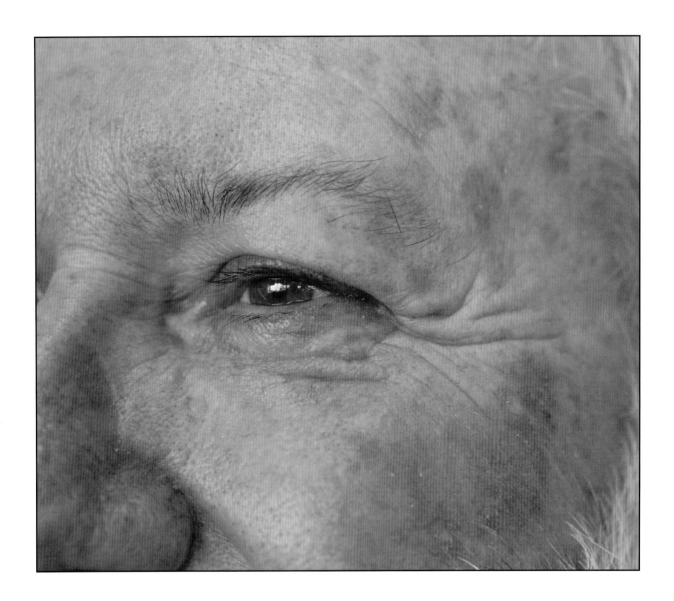

Kali Sulph (c)

This man's face, with brown spots on the temples, shows a Kali Sulph deficiency. He also has a chronic redness of the area below the eye – a Nat Sulph deficiency. The area above the nose has the large pores of a Nat Mur deficiency. The crow's-feet of the outer eye also indicate a severe Calc Fluor deficiency.

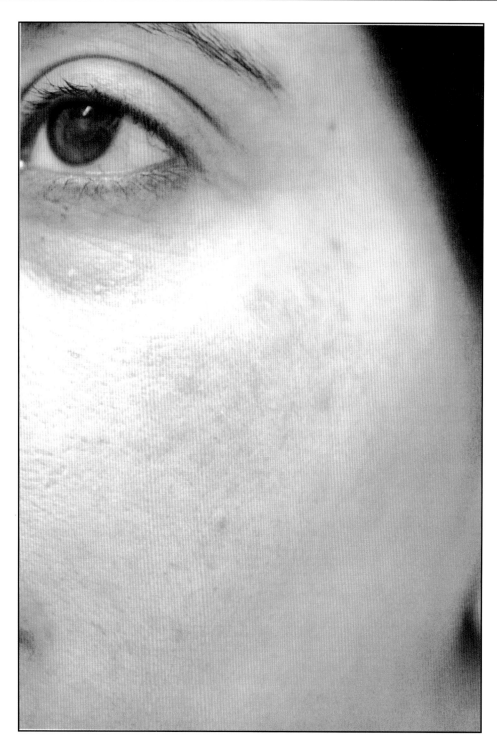

Kali Sulph (d)

This woman's face shows an aggressive brown spots (or melasma) that showed up after taking birth-control pills. This is a Kali Sulph deficiency caused by estrogen imbalance, and may also indicate weak liver function. Under the eye we see some large pores, typical of a Nat Mur deficiency.

and unseen elements. Nitrogen gas is mineral in solution, or ultimate potency.

Oil is made by the union of the sulphate of potassium (Kali Sulph), with albuminoids (proteins) and aerial elements. The first element that is disturbed in the organism of those born in the celestial sign Virgo is oil; this break in the function of oil shows that there is a deficiency in potassium sulphate, known in the pharmacy as Kali Sulph.

Virgo is represented in the human body by the stomach and bowels, the laboratory in which food is consumed as fuel to set free the minerals, in order to that they may enter the blood through the mucous membrane absorbents.

The letter X in Hebrew is Samech or Stomach. This "X," or cross, means crucifixion, or change-transmutation.

Virgo people are discriminating, analytical and critical.

The governing planet of this sign is Mercury. The gems associated with Virgo are pink jasper and hyacinth, and the astral colors are gold and black.

In the system of Biblical alchemy, Virgo is represented by Joseph, the twelfth son of Jacob and means "to increase power," or "son of the right hand."

The thirteenth child of Jacob, the Circle, is Benjamin; see Chapter 35 of Genesis. Virgo corresponds with the New Testament disciple Bartholomew.

CHAPTER 10

Mag Phos

This cell salt may be made by mixing phosphate of soda with sulphate of magnesia. It is found chiefly in the white fibers of nerves and muscles. The tissues of nerves and muscles are composed of many very fine threads or strands of different colors, each acting as a special telegraph wire, each one having a certain conductive power or quality, i.e., special chemical affinity – for certain organic substances, fatty acids and proteins, through and by which the organism is materialized and the process or operations of life are carried on. The imagination might easily conceive the idea that these delicate infinitesimal fibers are strings of the human harp, and that molecular minerals are the fingers of infinite energy, striking notes of some Divine anthem.*

The white fibers of nerves and muscles need the dynamic action of Mag Phos (also known as magnesia- or magnesium phosphate), especially to keep them in proper tune or function, for, by its chemical action on albumen, the special fluid for white nerve or muscle fiber is formed. When the supply of this salt falls below the standard, cramps, sharp shooting pains, or some spasmodic condition prevails. Such symptoms are simply calls of nature for more magnesia.

The human body is composed of perfect principles – gases, minerals, molecules or atoms; but these builders of flesh and bone are not always properly adjusted. The planks of bricks used in building houses may be endlessly diversified in arrangement and yet be perfect material. Therefore, we must conclude that symptoms of disease are dispatches sent to the brain (the throne of understanding) calling for the worker, the builder, needed to carry on life's work in flesh. Cases of chorea – involuntary limb movements (St. Vitus's dance) – are cured by the proper use of magnesia phosphate. This salt is the great remedy for nearly all heart troubles, except embolus (blood clots). (See Kali Mur)

*This complete introductory section is adapted from:
The Chemistry and Wonders of the Human Body by Dr. George Carey.

The white fibers in the delicate strands that compose the tissue of nerves are controlled by the molecules of magnesia; when these workers are deficient in amount, these live wires contract or cramp up in knots (of course infinitely small), the effect of which is a sharp shooting pain, as in so-called neuralgia, or sciatica. The word "neuralgia" is from (a) Latin for "nerves" (b) Greek for "pain," and therefore simply means "nerve pain." English expresses the effect quite as well as other languages. But the idea generally prevails that neuralgia means a thing unknown and indefinable that causes the pain, and that the name of this unknown thing is neuralgia.

The pain is simply a dispatch, or words, asking for magnesia phosphate. A deficiency of this salt in the muscular and nerve tissue of the walls of the stomach causes contraction (cramps), which reduces the cavity of the stomach. In order to meet this condition and prevent a collapse, such as is formed by a natural chemical process from material at hand and by expansion, Magnesia Phosphate produces a counter force that wards off more serious results. Magnesia Phosphate relieves such conditions immediately, thus demonstrating the theory that to supply the deficient tissue-builder is the natural method of cure. The phosphate of lime (Calc Phos) often supplements magnesia (Mag Phos).

This wonderful salt is the true antispasmodic remedy. It has cured cases of chorea in from 2-4 weeks. For all heart troubles caused by distension of the cardiac portion of the stomach, thus interfering with the action of the heart, it is the sovereign remedy. Dr. Boericke, one of the leading homeopathic physicians of the Pacific Coast, says, "Magnesia Phosphate is a magnificent remedy in all spasmodic diseases."

It is plainly evident that the wonderful fluids of the human body are manufactured in the chemical laboratory of the organism. The particles of magnesia evidently contain within themselves the power and potency to create the white-fiber nerve fluid by using albuminous (protein) substances as a basis, and then calling to its aid the spirit of life, oxygen. Each one of the inorganic salts knows how to make some fluid or tissue of the human machine. "And the tree bore twelve manner of fruits and its leaves were for the healing of the nations." (Revelations, 8:2)

Like the phosphate of potash (Kali Phos), Mag Phos is a nerve and brain salt, and when we consider the wonders of the brain and its marvelous mechanism, we must recognize the great importance of the wizard workmen that labor for three score and ten years without an instant of rest.

MATERIA MEDICA FOR MAG PHOS

Adapted from: *The Biochemic System of Medicine, Materia Medica* by Dr. George Carey

Molecules of magnesium phosphate (Mag Phos) are found chiefly in the white fibers of the nerves and muscles. Nerves and muscles are composed of many strands of fibers of different colors, each one acting as a special telegraph wire; each one having a conductive power or special affinity for certain organic and inorganic principles, and performing its varied functions through the operation of natural law. The white fibers are controlled by the molecular action of the magnesia cell salt.

When a deficiency in this salt occurs, these white fibers contract and produce a condition called "spasms," or "cramps." This symptom of cramps is merely the body's method of announcing a lack of magnesium phosphate, and showing the location where the deficiency has occurred. For convenience of description, different names are given to cramps and spasms in various parts of the body, but they are nevertheless all essentially the same, the result of a lack of magnesium phosphate.

When a deficiency of magnesium phosphate occurs in the muscular tissue of the walls of the stomach, the white fibers draw up, contract, and reduce the cavity of the stomach. Now, in order to meet this condition and prevent a collapse, gas is formed by a natural process from the material at hand, and by expansion produces a counter force. Magnesia phosphate relieves such conditions almost instantly.

The only exception to this rule of speedy cures by administering this remedy where the blood has furnished calcium phosphate as a substitute, in an effort to supply the deficiency. Calcium phosphate more nearly corresponds to magnesium phosphate than any other salt; therefore, when magnesium phosphate does not act very promptly, calcium phosphate should be given, in order to overcome the deficiency of that salt which has been caused in the blood.

Magnesia phosphate is the true antispasmodic remedy. It has cured cases of chorea (involuntary limb movement) or St. Vitus's dance, in from 2-4 weeks. For all heart troubles, so called, caused by a distention of the cardiac portion (upper valve) of the stomach, and thus interfering with the action of the heart, it is the sovereign remedy.

But the question will arise: How can molecules of a certain mineral salt supply a certain white nerve or muscle fluid? There is certainly a difference between the particles of an inorganic salt and the fluid that controls white fibers. To answer these questions, and try to make the matter clear to the minds of everybody, is the object of these short articles. It is quite evident that the fluid in question is manufactured in the physiology of the body.

The particles of magnesium phosphate simply contain within themselves the power – the potency – to create this muscle and nerve fluid by uniting with protein as the basic organic material, then calling to its aid the spirit of life, oxygen. Each inorganic salt knows how to make some constituent of the human organism.

Characteristic Indications

(Note: The remedies in parentheses are support for Mag Phos.)

Mental symptoms – Illusions of the senses and mental disorders. Mag Phos is closely allied with Kali Phos, as the latter acts upon the gray nerve fibers, while the former acts upon the white nerve fibers; these being so closely connected, it is evident that a molecular disturbance in one of them will be apt to cause a disturbance in the other, therefore, the characteristic indications of the two salts may, in some cases, be somewhat similar.

Head – Headache of the nervous character, with illusions of sight. Headaches, with sharp, shooting, darting, intermittent and spasmodic pain. Headache with chilly sensations, especially up and down the spine. **Neuralgia of head**, when the pain is sharp (Ferrum Phos). All pain when heat relieves and cold aggravates. Excruciating pains in the head, rheumatic or neuralgic. Pain in nape of neck of a sharp character. **Trembling and involuntary shaking of the head** (Kali Phos).

Eyes – Drooping of the eyelids (Kali Phos). Contracted pupils. Sparks, colors before the eyes. Illusions of the sense of sight. Sensitiveness to light, diplopia (double vision), spectra, etc. **Spasmodic stitching of the eyelids** (Calc Phos). Neuralgic pains in the eyes. Squinting. Calc Phos should be used externally and internally in most diseases of the eye; will act better if applied hot. Great pain in the eyes, with flow of tears requires Nat Mur. Dullness of sight from weakness of the optic nerve (Kali Phos).

Ears – Dullness of hearing, from disease of the auditory nerve fibers. **Earache, when of a purely nervous or spasmodic character**, heat relieves, all pains worse from cold.

Nose – "Loss of sense of smell, or perversion of the sense of smell, under certain conditions, not connected with cold; a course of this remedy" (Schuessler).

Face – Neuralgic pains of the face, of a shifting, shooting, darting, spasmodic character. Pains, lightning-like, worse to the touch and by cold; relieved by warm applications. Face ache, of a rheumatic character. Face ache (facial neuralgia) with flow of tears requires Nat Mur (if inflammatory, Ferrum Phos). Pains worse in cold air, better in warm room.

Mouth – Twitching of the mouth and lips, spasmodic. Tetanic spasms (continuous steady contractions). **Spasmodic stammering**; speaks slowly and begins speaking with the teeth closed (if nervous, Kali Phos). Lockjaw, should also be rubbed into the gums very frequently, internally, in hot water.

Teeth – Convulsions, cramps, etc., during dentition (alternate Calc Phos). Toothache, sharp, shooting, rheumatic and spasmodic pain, when heat relieves. If cold relieves, Ferrum Phos is the remedy, as it indicates an inflammatory condition of the nerve or some of the adjacent tissues. Teeth sensitive to the cold air or to touch. **Toothache, when associated with neuralgia of the face**, heat relieves, pains darting, intermittent and change about. In toothache, if Mag Phos fails, or the tooth is badly decayed, give Calc Phos.

Throat – Spasms of the throat, spasmodic closing of the windpipe. **Choking on attempting to swallow**. Spasmodic cough. Constricted feeling of the throat. Closing of the larynx by spasm or cramp. Shrill voice coming on suddenly when speaking or singing, caused by spasm of the windpipe (Kali Phos).

Gastric symptoms – Neuralgia of stomach; tongue clean, pain relieved by heat or pressure. Spasm of the stomach, when the pain is constricted or griping. Indigestion, when food causes griping; tongue clean (Calc Phos, Ferrum Phos). Hiccough. Vomiting, when caused by excessive pain or constriction of muscles of stomach. **Pain is remittent and spasmodic**. Belching of gas with short, sharp, nipping pain; drinking hot water relieves; worse from drinking acid or cold drinks.

Abdomen and stool – Dysentery (frequent watery, bloody, mucus-like stools), when accompanied by sharp griping pains in the abdomen, which are relieved by warmth, rubbing or pressure (Kali Mur). Remittent and spasmodic pain. Colic of infants, with screaming and drawing up of legs. Gnawing pains in the bowels, with belching of wind. **Bloating of the abdomen** with passing of flatus (gas). Griping pain in abdomen, with watery diarrhea, stools expelled with force. Hemorrhoids, with cutting darting pains, very severe. Pain in the rectum and abdomen.

In all cases of diarrhea, dysentery, neuralgia and inflammation of the bowels, copious injections of hot water should be given frequently; it will cleanse the unhealthy membrane, restore normal absorption, relax the abdominal muscles, wonderfully relieve pain and greatly aid in the restoration of the patient. Hot or cold applications should also be used. – Chapman

Urinary organs – Spasmodic retention of the urine (alternate Ferrum Phos). **Spasm of the bladder** and urethra, with **painful straining when urinating** (Ferrum Phos, Kali Phos). Pain when passing gravel (kidney stones)(Nat Sulph).

Male sexual organs – Stricture (constriction or narrowing) resulting from gonorrhea; sharp, spasmodic pains in the urethra.

Female sexual organs – Dysmenorrhea (menstrual colic), at the time to relieve the pain (Kali Phos). As a preventive, Ferrum Phos. Very severe pain, of "labor-like character," heat generally relieves. **Neuralgia of the ovaries**, apply hot local applications also. Menstrual colic, when membranes are thrown off, or the discharge is stringy or fibrous. Vaginismus (Ferrum Phos). Pain preceding the monthly flow.

Pregnancy – Labor pains, when they are spasmodic, or with cramps in the legs and spasmodic stitching. Excessive expulsive efforts. Convulsions (*see* Kali Phos).

Respiratory organs – Asthma, with belching of gas, pain in the chest, and constrictive cough, must sit up (give the remedy in hot water). Spasmodic cough, coming in fits or paroxysms, without expectoration. Sudden, shrill voice. Sharp pains in the chest, shortness of breath (Ferrum Phos). Whooping cough (Kali Mur). Must be given persistently in chronic cases. Spasm of the glottis. **Convulsive fits of coughing, with constriction of the chest** and little or no expectoration. Spasmodic coughing at night, worse on lying down.

Circulatory organs – Neuralgic spasms of the breast. When pain is severe in any organ, the remedy should be given in hot water, and very frequently doses.

Back and extremities – Pains in the back and extremities, of a neuralgic character, very sharp, darting, or remittent. Pain in small of back and neck, heat relieves. Convulsions, with stiffness of the limbs, clenched fingers (Calc Phos). Painful joints. **Neuralgia of the limbs.** Violent pains in rheumatism of the joints. Local applications. Sciatic rheumatism, with violent pains. **Shooting sensation in the limbs resembling electric shocks.** Power of motion deficient.

Nervous symptoms – Trembling and involuntary motion of the hands. Paralysis agitans (Parkinson's-like) (Kali Phos). Involuntary shaking of the head. **Epilepsy, from any cause**, for spasm (Kali Mur, chief remedy for the disease). Chorea. Lockjaw, frequent doses in hot water; also rub it into the gums. Compare with Kali Phos in all nervous diseases. Writer's cramp. Cramps in the limbs at night. **Patient is tired and exhausted**, from insufficient nutrition of the nerve tissues (Kali Phos). Want of sensibility.

Tissues – Spasms and neuralgic pains in any tissue, due to a deficiency of unequalization of the Mag Phos molecules.

Febrile conditions – Nervous chills, with chattering of the teeth (Kali Phos). Fever, when chills and cramps are present (Ferrum Phos). Intermittent fever, with cramps of the calves of limbs. Chills run up and down the spine.

Sleep – Yawning, with spasmodic straining of the lower jaw, sometimes throwing the jaw out of its socket. Drowsiness.

Modalities – All the symptoms of this remedy are relieved by heat, pressure and rubbing, and are aggravated by cold, cold air, drafts, etc. If practical, hot applications should always be used when this remedy is exhibited.

"THE INORGANIC SUBSTANCES IN THE BLOOD AND TISSUES ARE SUFFICIENT TO HEAL ALL DISEASES WHICH ARE CURABLE AT ALL."

– DR. SCHUESSLER

FACIAL SIGNS OF MAG PHOS DEFICIENCY

Magnesium red is the bright dynamic red without any other mixtures. This pattern shows an inner heat and the outer skin feels cool. (The Ferrum Phos red shows external heat and an inner cool.) The facial redness can come and go.

Flushing red comes and goes with stress or shame, embarrassment, or other emotions. It only appears in times of tension.

Constant red. We see a constant red appearance when the magnesium is strong enough. The redness appears opposite of the nasal wings in a round pattern up to 2 inches across. This is often seen in people who rarely eat fresh foods, or in girls in early menstruation.

Mag Phos has to do with the condition of the nerves. In stress conditions, red spots can appear anywhere on the cheeks or upper chest and neckline. These spots are most often seen in women.

Some people turn red after eating. It can be a colon weakness of Ferrum Phos deficiency or most likely a Mag Phos deficiency that shows up in the face. If the back of the hand is hot, then it is a Ferrum Phos deficiency.

Many people's faces turn red after alcohol consumption. The alcohol enlarges the arteries. If the enlargement of the arteries becomes too much, then it could be a Ferrum Phos problem. One could also use Nat Sulf to protect the liver.

THERAPEUTIC INDEX FOR MAG PHOS

Adapted from: *Therapeutic Index* (1890) by Dr. W. H. Schuessler

Back, pains in, very vivid, darting, boring, shifting about, and remittent (returning).
Cholera, cramps (severe colon).
Chorea, spasmodic, involuntary limb movements, or St. Vitus's dance.
Chromatopsia, spasmodic vision of rainbow colors.
Colic, flatulent, of children, with drawing up of legs.
Colic, forcing the patient to bend double (Colocynthis), which is eased by friction, warmth, and eructations (belching).
Colic in umbilical region (belly button), forcing the patient to bend forward (Colocynthis).
Colic, remittent (repeating indigestion).
Cough, spasmodic, coming in fits, paroxysms.
Cough, true spasmodic.
Cramp of the legs, or indeed in any part of the body.
Cramp, spasm of the larynx.
Diplopia, seeing double, an affection of the eye.
Dysentery, with crampy pain, eased by bending double, by warmth or friction.
Eczema, better, white scaly; often as second remedy.
Enuresis (bed wetting), involuntary flow of urine at night, if arising from nerve irritation.
Epigastric (abdominal) pains, nipping, griping, with short belching of wind, giving no relief.
Epigastric spasms, with clean tongue, feeling of crampy tight lacing.
Epilepsy, without rush of blood to head, nor the characteristics calling for Kali Phos.
Face-aches (Trigeminal neuralgia – either neuralgic or rheumatic), stinging, shooting, darting about, and remittent.
Glottis (throat), spasm of the.
Headaches, very excruciating, with tendency to spasmodic symptoms.
Headaches, (neuralgic, rheumatic) shooting or stinging, shifting and intermittent.
Intermittent fever, with cramp of the calves.
Labor pain, spasmodic, with cramp in legs.
Laryngismus stridulus, cramp or spasm of the larynx.
Limbs, pain in (neuralgic, rheumatic), very vivid, darting about, shifting and remittent.
Menstrual-colic; the chief remedy in ordinary cases.

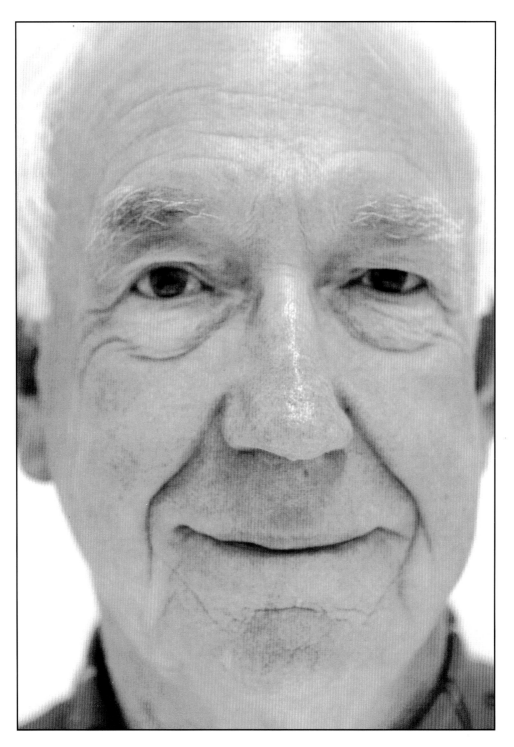

Mag Phos (a)

This man has the overall red face of a severe Mag Phos deficiency. He also has large eye bags, indicative of Nat Sulph deficiency. The chin shows a Nat Phos deficiency. The shiny forehead points out a Silicea deficiency.

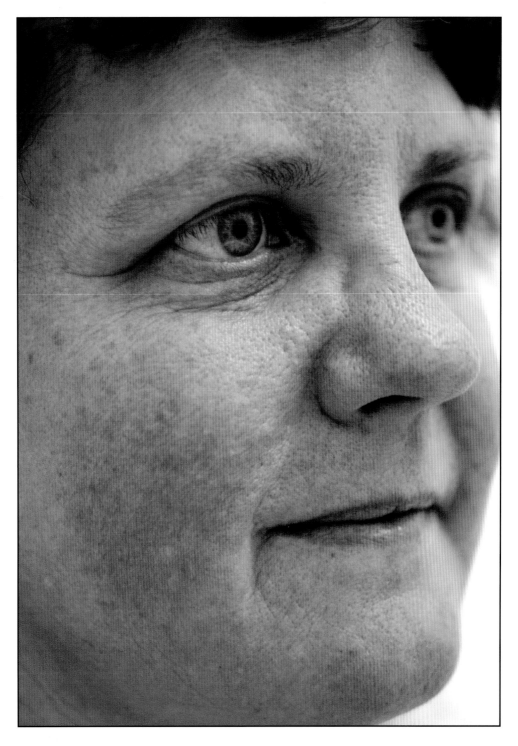

Mag Phos (b)

This woman's red face is the sign of a severe Mag Phos deficiency. The dark circles under the eye is a Ferrum Phos deficiency sign. There is a waxy appearance indicative of Calc Phos deficiency.

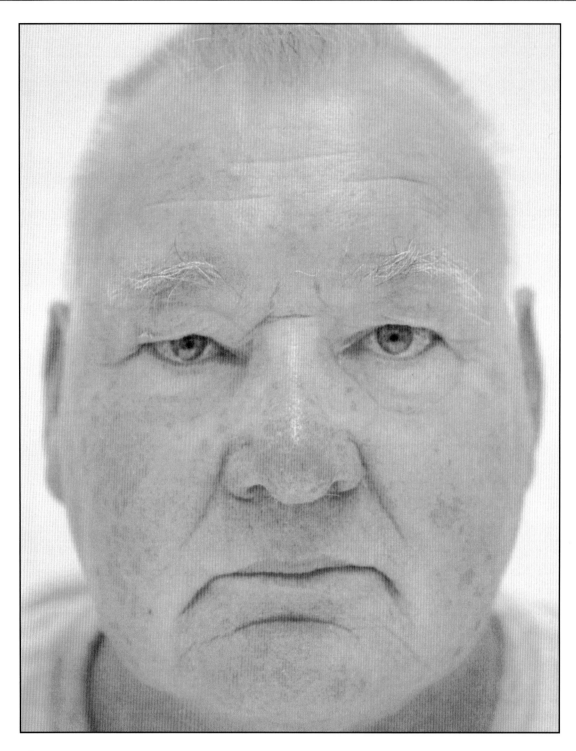

Mag Phos (c)

This man has a chronic red face, showing a severe Mag Phos deficiency. The nose is overlain with the deeper red of a Nat Sulph deficiency, which also includes lower swollen eye-bags. There are some subtle brown spots of a Kali Sulph deficiency.

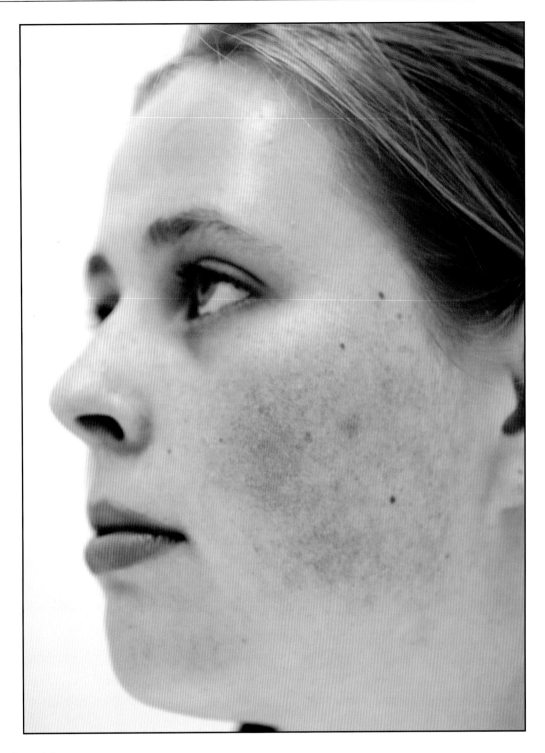

Mag Phos (d)

This woman has juvenile diabetes. Such cases often exhibit the red cheeks of Mag Phos deficiency. Under stress, the cheeks get redder, which is a characteristic of this deficiency. There is an overlay of brown spots, showing a Kali Sulph deficiency. Kali Sulph supports good liver function, and many diabetics are challenged by a poor liver.

Nape of neck, pains in, very vivid, shooting, boring, shifting, and remittent.

Photopsia, seeing sparks before the eye.

St Vitus's dance. (Involuntary limb spasms)

Stricture, spasmodic, of the bladder.

Teething cramps (convulsions) without fever.

Tetanus (lockjaw).

Toothache (neuralgic, rheumatic) very vivid, eased by warmth.

Tonic spasms (steady-tension muscle lock-up).

ASTROLOGY OF MAG PHOS
Leo: The Heart of the Zodiac
July 22 to August 22

Adapted from: *Cell Salts of Salvation* by Dr. George Carey

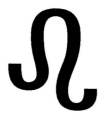 The Sun overflows with divine energy. It is the "brewpot" that forever filters and scatters the "Elixir of Life." Those born while the Sun is passing through Leo, July 22 to August 22, receive the heart vibrations, or pulses, of the Grand Man, or "Circle of Beasts." All the blood in the body passes through the heart and the Leo native is the recipient of every quality and possibility contained in the great "Alchemical Vase," the "Son of Heaven."

The impulsive traits of Leo people are symbolized in the pulse, which is a reflex of heart-throbs. The astronomer, by the unerring law of mathematics applied to space, proportion, and the so-far-discovered wheels and cogs of the uni-machine, can tell where a certain planet must be located before the telescope has verified the prediction. So the astro-biochemist knows there must of necessity be a blood mineral and tissue builder to correspond with the materialized angel of the circle of the zodiac.

The Mag Phos, in biochemic therapeutics, is the remedy for all spasmodic impulsive symptoms. This salt supplies the deficient worker or builder in such cases and thus restores normal conditions. A lack of muscular force, or nerve vigor, indicates a disturbance in the operation of the heart cell-salt, magnesia phosphate, which gives the "Lion's spring" or impulse to the blood that throbs through the heart.

Leo is ruled by the Sun, and the children of that celestial sign are natural sun worshipers.

Gold must contain a small percent of alloy or base metal before it can be used commercially. Likewise the "Gold of Ophir" – Sun's rays, or vibration – must contain a high potency of the earth salt, magnesia, in order to be available for use in bodily function. Thus, through the chemical action of the inorganic (mineral and water) in the organic, Sun's rays and ether, does the volatile become fixed, and the word becomes flesh.

Leo people consume their birth salts more rapidly than they consume any of the other salts of the blood; hence are often deficient in magnesium. Crude magnesia is too coarse to enter the blood through the delicate mucus membrane absorbents, and must be prepared according to the biochemic method before taken to supply the blood.

In Biblical alchemy, the eleventh child of Jacob, Dinah, represents Leo and means "judged." Gems of Leo are ruby and diamond, and the astral colors are red and green. In the New Testament, Simon is the Leo disciple.

CHAPTER 11

Nat Mur

Nat Mur is also called sodium chloride. A combination of sodium and chlorine forms the mineral known as common salt. This mineral absorbs water. The circulation or distribution of water in the human organism is due to the chemical action of the molecules of sodium of chloride. This inorganic cell salt is the bearer and distributor of water.*

Water constitutes over 70 percent of the human body; therefore, the carriers of water must be in like proportion. There is more sodium chloride in the ashes of a cremated body than any of the twelve mineral salts, except phosphate of lime (Calc Phos), which composes 57 percent of bone structure.

Through its affinity for water, this salt assists in carrying on the process of life in the human organism as well as in all vegetable tissue. When there is a deficiency in the molecules of the water-bearer, i.e., salt, the molecular continuity of water is broken and, as a result, too much water will appear at a certain point and corresponding dryness or lack or water at other places. Example: watery discharge from nasal passages and constipation of the bowels.

Sunstroke and delirium tremens (alcohol-withdrawal shakes) are caused by a break in the supply of this salt, which causes water to press or crowd the membranes of the cerebellum (lower brain), and thus prevent the magnetic vibrations from the cerebrum (upper brain) from passing to the solar plexus, or central brain.

Crude soda (sodium) cannot be taken up by mucus membrane absorbents and carried into circulation. The sodium molecules found in the blood have been received from vegetable tissue that drew these salts from the soil in high potency. The mineral, or cell salts, can also be prepared and are prepared in biochemic or homeopathic potency as the trituration of nature's laboratory in the physiology of plant growth, and then thoroughly

*This complete introductory section is adapted from:
The Chemistry and Wonders of the Human Body by Dr. George Carey.

mixed with sugar of milk and pressed into tablets ready to be taken internally to supply deficiencies in the human organism. A lack of the proper amount of these basic mineral salts, twelve in number, is the cause of all so-called disease. Common table salt does not enter the blood, being too coarse to enter the delicate tubes of mucus membrane absorbent, but this salt does distribute water along the intestinal tract.

Professor Leibig says in his *Chemical Letters* that muriatic acid (hydrochloric acid), when diluted a thousand-fold with water, dissolves with ease at the temperature of the body, fibrin and gluten, and that this solvent power does not increase, but diminishes if the proportion of acid in the dilution be increased.

Air contains 78 percent of nitrogen gas, believed by scientists to be mineral in ultimate potency. Minerals are formed by the precipitation of nitrogen gas. Differentiation is attained by the proportion of oxygen and aqueous vapor (hydrogen) that united with nitrogen.

A deficiency in Nat Mur causes the water in the blood serum to become inert and non-functional. By its affinity for water, sodium chloride assists in the biological operation of blood and tissue.

As will be seen in Chapter 13, Nat Sulph eliminates an excess of water in the blood and thus regulates the supply; while Nat Mur properly distributes water in the physiology of animal or vegetable forms.

Materia Medica of Nat Mur

Adapted from: *The Biochemic System of Medicine, Materia Medica* by Dr. George Carey

With the exception of the phosphate of lime (Calc Phos), the human system contains more sodium chloride than any other inorganic salt. The reason for this may be readily understood when we realize that our bodies are about 70 percent water, which, in the absence of sodium chloride, would be inert and useless. It is the power that this salt has to use water that renders it of any value to man. The same principle holds good in plants and vegetable life.

Nat Mur uses water to build up and carry on the functions of life, and also as a vehicle to eliminate waste substances. Any deficiency in this cell salt at once causes a disturbance of the water in the human organism, because it has lost that element which renders it fit to perform its allotted task. In sunstroke, a deficiency in sodium chloride allows the moisture to be drawn from other parts, especially the nape of the neck, and causes a pressure against the base of the brain, producing dangerous and sometimes fatal results. The above named salt relieves the unpleasant condition called sunstroke, surely and quickly.

In delirium tremens the continuity of water is broken up due to a deficiency of sodium chloride molecules, and the symptoms incident to this disease follow. Very severe cases of delirium tremens have been relieved in one hour by administering frequent doses of this remedy.

People will wish to know more than the mere fact that a certain agent has curative properties; they will demand to know "how and why." And if the remedy is the true one, the "how and why" can always be explained.

It is necessary to make clear the modus operandi of the twelve inorganic salts; to show that each one has a special building or creative power. This salt may be compared to a brick mason or carpenter. The brick mason has the power to build up a brick wall when he is supplied with brick and mortar. So the carpenter can create a wooden structure when lumber and other material necessary for the work is furnished. The carpenter is the workman, or vitalizer, of the inert organic material and possesses the creative power to produce a building. So the inorganic salts possess the creative power to make something out of organic matter; and thus the chemistry of life goes on.

Characteristic Indications

(Note: The remedies in parentheses are support for Nat Mur.)

Mental symptoms – Delirium at any time, with muttering and wandering, when the tongue has a frothy appearance, or is dry and parched. Stupor and sleepiness. Low delirium in typhoid or typhus fevers. Delirium tremens; this salt is the chief remedy to overcome the dryness which exists in the brain (Kali Phos). Melancholy, hopeless, with dejected spirits. Despondent moods, with constipation or excess of watery symptoms, weeps easily.

Head – Chief remedy in sunstroke; this disease, like delirium tremens, is due to an excessive dryness of the tissue of the brain, owing to a disturbance of the sodium chloride molecules. Headaches, with dryness of some of the mucus membranes and excessive secretion from others. Headaches, with constipation. **Headaches, with profusion of tears** or frothy coating on the tongue; hopeless, dejected spirits. Headaches, with vomiting of frothy, watery phlegm. Headaches of girls in puberty; patient is dull and listless. Dull, heavy, hammering headaches, with drowsiness and unrefreshing sleep. Eruptions of the scalp, with watery contents. Dandruff. White scales on the scalp (Kali Sulph, Kali Mur).

Eyes – Neuralgic pains in the eyes, with flow of tears (Mag Phos). Flow of tears from the eyes, when associated with fresh colds in the head. Weak eyes, with tears when going into cold air or when the wind strikes the eyes. All eye affections with flow of tears. Granulated eyelids, with or without secretion of tears (Ferrum Phos, Kali Mur). Blisters, on the cornea (Kali Mur); should also be syringed daily with a solution of the salt to produce absorption of the spot. Stoppage of the tear duct from colds. Pain in the eyes, with tears, recurring daily at certain times. Scrofulous conditions of the eyes, thick lids, acrid, smarting secretions, with tears. Muscular asthenopia (weakness) (Mag Pos). Conjunctivitis, with mucus secretions and lachrymation (tears).

Ears – Deafness from swelling of the Eustachian tubes (Kali Mur, Kali Sulph). Ear affections, with excessive secretion of saliva or characteristic discharge from the ears.

Nose – Fresh colds, with discharge of clear, watery, transparent mucus and sneezing. Dropping of watery, salty secretion from the posterior nares (Calc Phos). Chronic catarrh of anemic persons, with salty mucus. Hay fever, influenza, with sneezing and watery discharges from eyes and nose. Coryza (running cold), with watery, slimy discharge. Loss of smell, with dryness and rawness of the pharynx. Bleeding of the nose in anemic persons; the blood is thin and watery (Ferrum Phos). Excessive dryness with tendency to form scales or crusts in the nose.

Face – Face ache (trigeminal neuralgia), with constipation; tongue covered with a clear mucus, slime and frothy bubbles at its edge. Face ache, with vomiting of clear phlegm of water. Neuralgia of the face, with excessive discharge of clear mucus from the eyes (local application of the same). Whiskers fall out; if the watery symptoms correspond. **Perspiration on the face while eating.** Chlorosis (green face), sallow, dirty-looking.

Mouth – Excess of saliva, alone or during the course of any disease. Salivation. **Catarrhs** (mucus congestion) of the mouth and pharynx, **with watery, transparent, frothy, discharges** (clear thick mucus, Calc Phos). Aphthe (thrush), with flow of saliva (alternate Kali Mur). Swelling of glands under the tongue. Ranula (cyst under tongue). Inflammation of salivary glands when secreting excessive amount of saliva. **Constant spitting of frothy mucus.**

Teeth – Toothache, with excessive flow of tears or saliva. **Neuralgia of teeth** and facial nerves, with characteristic secretions. Teething in infants and drooling.

Throat – Inflammation of mucus lining of the throat, with characteristic watery secretions.

Uvula relaxed when there is much saliva (Calc Fluor, chief remedy). Goiter, with watery symptoms (Calc Phos, chief remedy). Sore throat, with excessive dryness or too much secretion of saliva. In **diphtheria**, when there is drowsiness, **watery stools**, flow of saliva or vomiting of water; face is puffy and pale. Mumps, when watery symptoms are present (Kali Mur, chief remedy for swelling). Thin neck, with chlorotic (anemic) conditions.

Gastric symptoms – All conditions and diseases of the stomach where excess of saliva or watery vomit is present; tongue has a clear, frothy, transparent coating. **Indigestion with watery vomiting** and salty taste in the mouth. Patient sometimes has a great **craving for salt or salty food**. Indigestion with pain in stomach and watery gathering in the mouth, sour or salt taste in mouth. Great thirst. Dyspepsia (poor digestion), with pain after eating, if watery symptoms are present. Vomiting of transparent, watery stringy mucus, or watery fluids and froth (not acid). Jaundice, with drowsiness and watery symptoms. Water brash (heartburn), not acid, frequently accompanied with constipation, from dryness of the intestines.

Abdomen and stool – Looseness of the bowels, with watery stools. Diarrhea, alternating with constipation. Constipation from dryness of the mucus membranes of the bowels, with watery secretion in other parts. **Constipation, with dull, heavy headache, profusion of tears**, or vomiting of frothy water. Stools are dry and often produce fissure in rectum, burning pain in rectum, or torn, bleeding, smarting feeling after stool. Constipation, with drowsiness and watery symptoms from eyes or mouth. Diarrhea, stool frothy, glairy (like egg-white) slime, **causing soreness and smarting**. Hemorrhoids, with constipation, caused from dryness of the bowels. Stinging piles (hemorrhoids). Weakness of bowels and muscles of the abdomen. An occasional injection of hot water, with Nat Mur, will be found very beneficial. Nat Mur not only controls the watery secre-

tions of the bowels but it has a stimulating effect and will strengthen the muscles of the viscera and abdomen.

Urinary organs – Catarrh of the bladder when secreting watery, transparent fluid. Polyuria (frequent urination). Cutting and burning after urinating. Diabetes insipidus (pituitary diabetes); great thirst and excessive flow of watery urine.

Male sexual organs – **Chronic gonorrhea, with transparent, watery, scalding slime**. Chronic syphilis, with serous discharge. Hydrocele (fluid collection in scrotum). Preputial edema (swelling of prepuce of the penis) (Nat Sulph). Discharge of watery urine

Female sexual organs – Gonorrhea and syphilis, with characteristic discharges, indicating this remedy. **Menstrual flow thin, watery blood**. Menstruation too late, accompanied with sadness, headache and weeping. Delayed menstruation in young girls, when there is headache, dullness and sadness, or when the person is emaciated or chlorotic (anemic, characterized by a green tint to the skin). Soreness and smarting in vagina after urinating. Itching of the vulva. Menses mixed with leucorrhoea; discharges are smarting, scalding and watery. Watery, slimy, excoriating leucorrhoea. Dryness of vagina; sexual connection causes great pain. Vaginal douches of about 4 teaspoons of salt to 1 quart of warm water, of much benefit. Smarting, burning, sticking pain in vagina; inflammation caused by dryness of mucus membrane.

Pregnancy – Vomiting of watery, frothy phlegm, not acid.

Respiratory organs – Asthma, with watery, frothy mucus (alternate Kali Phos for the breathing). Bronchitis; mucus frothy and watery, sometimes coughed up with difficulty. Acute inflammation of the windpipe, with characteristic expectoration, constant spitting of frothy water. **Edema of the lungs, with watery expectoration**, sometimes tasting salty. Catarrh of the bronchi, "winter cough," with characteristic symptoms (note appearance of tongue). Chronic coughs of consumptives (tuberculosis), with frothy discharges, salty taste. Cough, with headache and excessive lachrymation. Cough, with flow of tears and spurting of urine (Ferrum Phos). In whooping cough, note the expectoration. **Pneumonia, with characteristic expectoration and much loose, rattling phlegm in the chest** (Ant Tart); note also tongue symptoms. Pleurisy, when serous effusion has taken place. Hoarseness. Pain in chest from coughing (Ferrum Phos).

Circulatory organs – Palpitation of the heart, in anemic persons, with watery blood, or dropsical (puffy) swellings. Enlargement of the heart, with characteristic indications. Poor circulation, cold hands and feet (Calc Phos). Pulse rapid and intermittent; **pulsations of heart felt all over the body.** Blood thin and watery; will not coagulate.

Back and extremities – Weak and languid feelings, with drowsiness. Blisters on the hands or fingers, containing watery, serous fluid. **Involuntary movement of the legs;** fidgets; cannot sit still. Starting and jerking of limbs during sleep (Mag Phos). Rheumatic, gouty pains, if tongue and watery secretions correspond. Rheumatism of the joints; joints crack (Rhus Tox); note appearance of tongue and watery symptoms. Pains in the back and extremities; **backache relieved by lying on something hard.** Hangnails, when there is dryness of the skin. Rheumatic gout, coming on periodically. Feeling of coldness in the back.

Nervous symptoms – Neuralgic nerve pains, with flow of saliva or tears, or when recurring periodically (Mag Phos). Sensation of numbness in parts affected; spine, cannot bear to have it touched, oversensitive to pressure; paralytic pain in small of back. Neuralgia; pains shoot along the nerve fibers, but accompanied by flow of saliva or tears. Hysterical; feels worse in the morning or in cold weather. Hysterical spasms and debility. Restlessness and twitching of the muscles.

Skin – All skin diseases, where there is a watery exudation, or in excessive dryness of the skin. Eczema, with white scales; external applications also. **Eruptions of the skin, with watery contents;** note tongue and watery symptoms. Colorless, watery vesicles. Herpes in bend of knee. Herpetic eruptions on any part of the body, or occurring during course of a disease. Chafing of skin in small children with watery symptoms (alternate Nat Phos). White scales on the scalp (Kali Sulph, chief remedy). Warts in palms of hands. Hangnails. Stings of insects (Ledum); apply locally as soon as possible. Smallpox, with drowsiness and flow of saliva. Shingles, with characteristic symptoms calling for this remedy. Rupia (brown cone-like layers), blisters with watery contents. Intertrigo (see Glossary) between thighs and scrotum, with acrid and excoriating discharge. Scarlet fever with watery vomiting, drowsiness, twitchings. **Exudations** on the skin or mucus lining, after inflammations, when **watery and serous.** Blisters and blebs on the skin, with watery contents. **Nettle rash, with violent itching;** appears after becoming overheated, causing an unequalization of this salt. Nettle rash in intermittent fever. Eczema from eating too much salt. Chronic skin diseases, especially urticarious (rashy) and miliary (small, like millet seeds) eruptions.

Tissues – Dropsy (swelling) in any part of the body (Nat Sulph). Accumulations of serum or water in the areolar tissues (dark ring). Dryness of some of the mucus membranes, with excess of secretions of others. Anemic conditions, with thin, watery blood. Chlorotic (anemic) conditions; chlorosis, with dirty, torpid skin. Face pale and sallow, when watery symptoms are present. Effusions (breaking open), serous, poor in albumen, slimy, like boiled starch. Note also tongue and watery secretions. Chronic inflammation of lymphatic glands; with watery secretions from some of the membranes. Mumps. Emaciations, especially of the neck; acts upon cartilage, mucus, follicles, glands, etc. Emaciation while living well. Cachexia (emaciation) following ague (fever/chill) from excessive use of quinine. The **slimy, frothy appearance of the tongue, with watery secretions**, is the keynote for this remedy. It regulates the proper degree of moisture of solids and proper amount of water of the fluids in the organism.

Febrile conditions – In all kinds of fevers, when there are malignant symptoms, such as stupor, drowsiness, watery vomiting, twitching, etc. Typhoid, typhus, scarlet fevers, with the above symptoms. **intermittent fever, after the abuse of quinine**; living in damp regions or on newly-turned ground (in alternation with Nat Sulph, chief remedy). Chill coming on in the morning about 10 o'clock and continuing till noon, preceded by intense heat, increased headache and thirst, sweat weakening and sour, backache and headache, great languor, emaciated sallow complexion, and fever blisters on the lips. Profuse night-sweats; bathe once a day in salt water. Feeling of chilliness, especially in the back; watery saliva; full, heavy headache, increased thirst, etc.

Sleep – Excessive sleep, if traced to an excess of moisture in the brain. **Constant desire to sleep**, drowsy, dull and stupid, when accompanied by the characteristic symptoms of this salt. Natural amount of sleep does not refresh, patient feels tired and stupid in the morning.

Modalities – Symptoms are generally worse in the morning, in cold weather, or in a salty atmosphere; feels better in the evening. Complaints from excessive use of allopathic medications. Complaints coming at regular periods.

FACIAL SIGNS OF NAT MUR DEFICIENCY

Gelatinous appearance. One can see the trail of a snail, and that is the look. It is a moist appearance. It is often seen on the upper eyelid, best seen with the eyes closed. With a Nat Mur deficiency, the tears are salty and have deposits in the lower eyelashes. Just below the lower eyelash there can be a 2-3 millimeter stripe of gelatinous appearance. There may be a slimy eyelid border.

A Nat Mur deficiency is also seen as an inflamed eyelid border because of a malfunctioning sodium chloride intercellular exchange. It is often seen in chronic conditions.

Large pores are often seen on the nose, on the cheeks, on the chin or forehead, but can be seen anywhere on the face. Nat Mur can reduce or eliminate the appearance.

There is a phenomenon where a Nat Mur deficiency shows up as **redness on the hair border** on the forehead. This is a long-standing deficiency.

Dandruff is a sign which is not strictly seen on the face, but its effects are seen on the hair and clothing. The problem is an inner deficiency and outer measures (such as medicated shampoos, etc.) can be detrimental. This is where the skin is too dry and flakes off.

Dry skin is not only seen on the face but can be over the entire body. The forehead may be greasy even though the skin is dry.

Puffy cheeks. This is a rarer sign that is seen now and again. This looks like one is blowing an instrument, etc.

Spongy or bloated appearance. The facial appearance comes with the moisture in the skin, and the ability to retain it. The pores try to hold the water and swell in response. The face seems swollen. Alcohol intake is often the cause or a great contributor.

The ringing or noise in the nose is because of altered mucus membranes in the nose. This is another sign of a Nat Mur deficiency. There is dryness or congestion or there is a clear runny nose.

Sweat regulates the bodily temperature. The Nat Mur deficiency shows up in the body's production of too much or too little sweat.

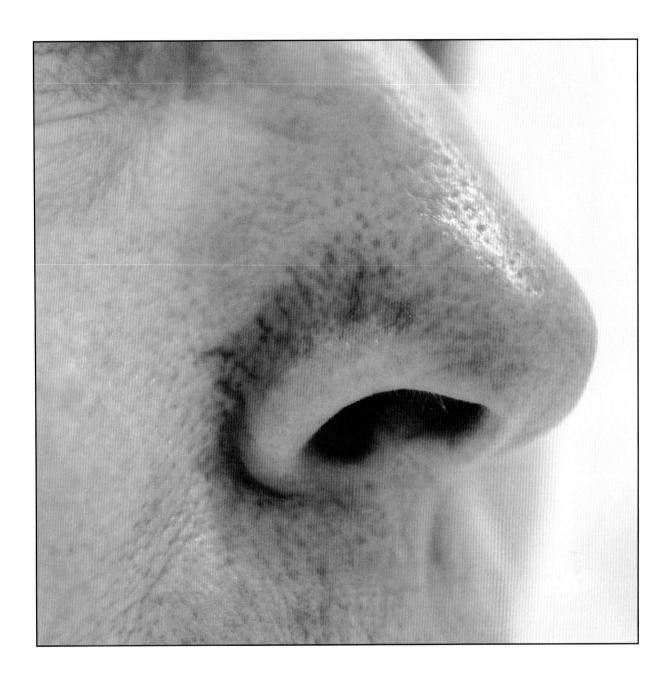

Nat Mur (a)

The shiny root of the nose shows the large pores of a severe Nat Mur deficiency. The corner of the eye has a dark black coloring – a Ferrum Phos deficiency sign. The overall redness illustrates a Mag Phos deficiency.

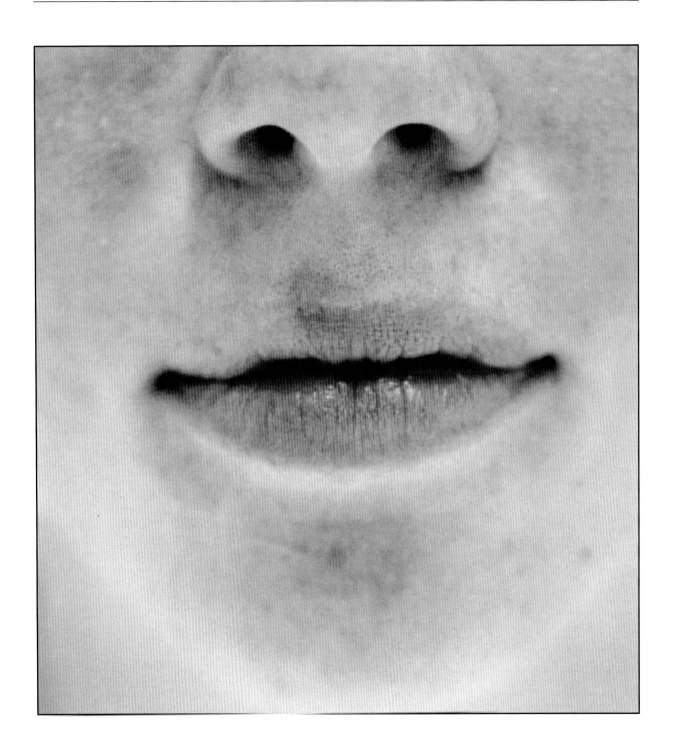

Nat Mur (b)

This woman has a fever blister on the upper lip characteristic of a Nat Mur deficiency. She also has a yellow coloring around the mouth, indicative of a Kali Sulph deficiency. The redness and pimples of the chin and cheeks are a Nat Phos deficiency.

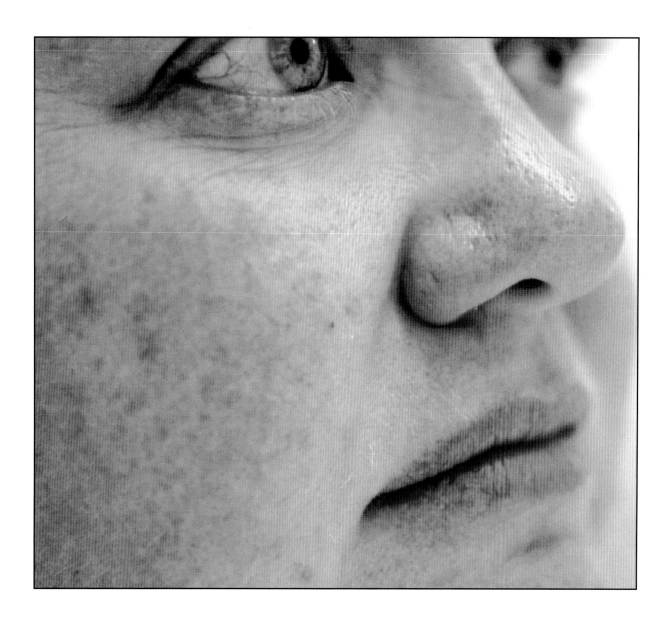

Nat Mur (c)

This woman's nose has the large pores of a Nat Mur deficiency. The cheeks show a Mag Phos deficiency symptom. She has yellow around her mouth, indicating a Kali Sulph deficiency. She has the dark brown-black circles of a Calc Fluor deficiency.

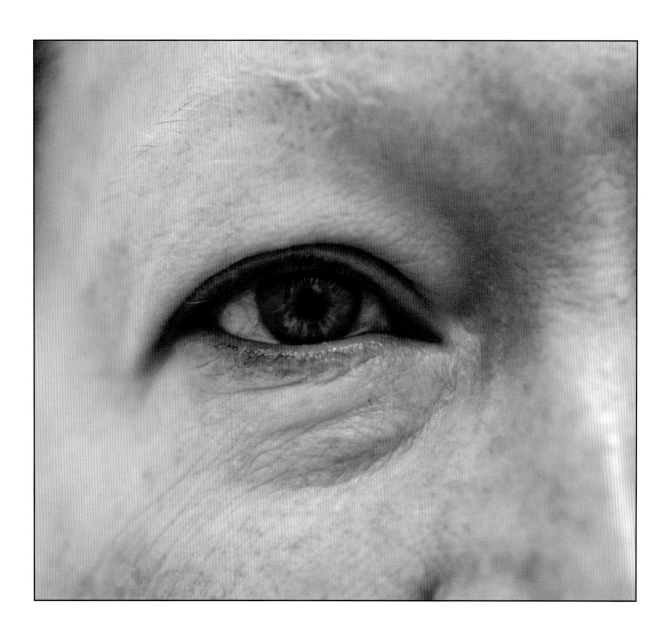

Nat Mur (d)

The photo of this eye shows a gelatinous shine in the eyelash area of the lower eyelid and large pores around the eyes. These are Nat Mur deficiency signs. The lower eyelid bags are signs of Nat Sulph deficiency.

THERAPEUTIC INDEX FOR NAT MUR

Adapted from: *Therapeutic Index* (1890) by Dr. W. H. Schuessler

Adynamic (weakness) conditions, with drowsiness, watery vomiting, etc.

Aphthae, thrush, with flow of saliva. (cankers)

Bronchitis, inflammation of the windpipe, after Kali Mur; if the loose rattling phlegm is coughed up with difficulty, and is frothy and clear.

Nat Mur Summary

ORGAN AND TISSUE AFFINITIES
Digestion, connective tissue, upper stomach, brain, blood, muscles, glands, skin, kidney, bladder.

MODALITIES
Symptoms worse < 9-11 a.m., sun, heat, physical exertion, talking, writing, reading, bread, noise, music.
Symptoms better > sweating, rest, open air, going without regular meals, deep breathing.

DEFICIENCY SYMPTOMS
Dandruff, dryness, loss of smell or taste, high blood pressure, cracking joints, sinus, must have sun glasses, can't cry in public, holds in old hurts.

DISEASE CONDITIONS
Depression, grief, herpes (facial or genital), infertility, M.S., sun problems, vaginal dryness, clear runny nasal or sinus discharges.

Catarrhs, chronic, of bloodless patients, mucus salty taste.

Chlorotic conditions, (anemia with green face) like "green sickness," if symptoms correspond to this remedy.

Constipation, chronic, the concurrent symptoms must decide this choice.

Coryza, with watery clear slimy discharges.

Cough, in consumption, chronic; watery symptoms.

Dandruff, scales, white, on scalp, with accompanying watery eruptions.

Deafness, from swelling of the tympanitic cavity, with corresponding symptoms.

Diarrhea, with transparent, glassy, slimy stools.

Diphtheria, if face is puffy and pale, with vomiting of watery fluid, and dryness of tongue, drowsiness of watery stools.

Eczema, white, scaly.

Edema of lungs, acute, serous, frothy secretions.

Eyes, discharge of clear mucus, and flow of tears.

Eyes, (neuralgic) pains, periodically appearing, with flow of tears.

Face ache (trigeminal neuralgia), with constipation, tongue showing a clear mucus, and little frothy bubbles at the edges of tongue.

Face ache, with vomiting of clear phlegm or water.

Fingers, blistering festers, watery bloody fluid, supposed to be caused by arsenical wallpapers.

Glands, chronic inflammation, with corresponding symptoms, excess of saliva, etc.

Glands lymphatic, chronic swelling, if with corresponding watery symptoms.

Gonorrhea, according to the characteristic secretions.

Headaches, with constipation, and tongue covered with a clear, slimy mucus, and frothy edges.

Headaches, with vomiting of transparent phlegm or water.

Hemorrhage, bleedings, blood pale red, thin, watery, not coagulating.

Herpes zoster, as second remedy.

Housemaid's knee, enlargement of bursa (joint sac), the chief remedy.

Hydrocele (testicular watery swelling).

Intertrigo, soreness of children, with watery symptoms.

Jaundice, according to the peculiar symptoms of this remedy.

Kidney, Bright's disease, with symptoms characteristic to the above remedy.

Knee, chronic swelling.

Leucorrhoea "Whites" (vaginal discharge) watery, scalding, irritating.

Lungs, inflammation of, if there is much loose, rattling phlegm, which has not been reabsorbed under Kali Mur, is coughed up with difficulty, and is clear and frothy.

Morning sickness with vomiting of watery, frothy phlegm.

Mumps, with much salivation.

Nettle rash, with accompanying watery symptoms.

Neuralgia, periodic, with great flow of saliva or tears (Merc Sol).

Orchitis (inflammation of testicles), after suppression of gonorrhea, if with characteristic secretions.

Pemphigus, blisters starting up on burning spots.

Polyuria, frequent urination, in diabetes (possible pituitary problem), if the symptoms correspond.

Rheumatic fever, after the second remedy, and where the characteristic symptoms indicate it.

Rheumatic, gouty pain, if symptoms correspond.

Rheumatism of the joints, chronic, if tongue or other symptoms correspond, and if joints crack.

Rupia, blistering, not pustular, eruptions in first stage.

Scarlet fever, with sopor (fatigue), twitchings, dryness of tongue, vomiting of watery fluids.

Secretions, if frothy, clear, slimy.

Secretions, if frothy, clear, white, like white of egg, or if like boiled starch.

Secretions on the skin, watery, not sticky, with other corresponding symptoms; else Nat Sulph.

Smallpox, with salivary flow, confluence of pustules, and spoor (drowsiness).

Stomachache, with much water (saliva) gathering in the mouth; if not curative, the tongue must be examined for Kali Sulph symptoms.

Sycosis (affection of the bearded part of the face), if the watery symptoms correspond.

Teething, with flow of saliva, much dribbling.

Throat, inflammation of the mucus lining, with transparent frothy mucus covering the tonsils.

Tongue, coating of, slimy and when small bubbles of frothy saliva cover the sides.

Toothache, with involuntary flow of tears.

Toothache, with great flow of saliva.

Typhoid conditions during the course of any fever, twitchings, with sopor, dryness of tongue, watery vomiting.

Vomiting of transparent, tough stringy mucus.

Vomiting of watery fluids (not acid).

Whooping cough, as third remedy.

Worms, (parasites) predisposition to, if with corresponding symptoms.

ASTROLOGY OF NAT MUR
Aquarius: The Sign of the Son of Man
January 20 to February 19

Adapted from: *Cell Salts of Salvation* by Dr. George Carey

O age of man: Aquarius,
Transmuter of all things base,
"Son of Man in the Heavens,"
With sun-illumined face.

Our journey was long and weary,
With pain and sorrow and tears,
But now at rest in thy kingdom,
We welcome the coming years.

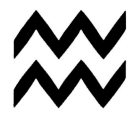Those born between the dates January 20 and February 19 are doubly blest, and babies to be born during that period for many years to come will be favored of the gods.

The Solar System has entered the "Sign of the Son of Man," Aquarius, where it will remain for over 2,000 years. According to planetary revolutions the Sun passes through Aquarius once every solar year; thus we have double influence of the Aquarius vibration from January 20 to February 19.

Air contains 78 percent of the nitrogen gas, believed by scientists to be mineral in ultimate potency. Minerals are formed by the precipitation of nitrogen gas. Differentiation is attained by the proportion of oxygen and aqueous vapor (hydrogen) that unites with nitrogen.

A combination of sodium and chlorine forms the mineral known as common salt. This mineral absorbs water. The circulation or distribution of water in the human organism is due to chemical action of the molecules of sodium chloride.

Aquarius is known in astrological symbol as "The Water Bearer." Sodium chloride, known as natrum muriaticum (Nat Mur), is also a bearer of water, and chemically corresponds with the zodiacal angel of Aquarius. The term "angle," or "angel," of the Sun may also be used, for the position of the Sun at birth largely controls the vibration of the blood. So, then, we have Nat Mur as the "birth salt" of Aquarius people.

The governing planets are Saturn and Uranus. The gems are sapphire, opal and turquoise, the astral colors are blue, pink and Nile green. Aquarius is an air-sign. In Bible alchemy, Aquarius represents Dan, the fifth son of Jacob, and means "judgment" or " he that judges." In the symbolism of the New Testament, Aquarius corresponds with the disciple James.

CHAPTER 12

Nat Phos

This alkaline cell salt is made from bone ash or by neutralizing orthophosphoric acid with carbonate of sodium. Nat Phos (also known as phosphate of sodium, or natrum phosphate) holds the balance between acids and normal fluids of the human body.*

Acid is organic and can be chemically split into two or more elements, thus destroying the formula that makes the chemical rate of motion called acid. Acid conditions are not due to an excess of acid in the blood, bile or gastric fluids. Supply the alkaline salt sodium phosphate, and acid will chemically change to normal fluids.

A certain amount of acid is necessary and always present in the blood, nerve, stomach and liver fluids. The apparent excess of acid is nearly always due to a deficiency in the alkaline, salt.

Acid, in alchemical lore, is represented as Satan (Saturn) while sodium phosphate (Nat Phos) symbolizes Christ (Venus). An absence of the Christ principle gives license to Satan to run riot in the Holy Temple. The advent of Christ drives the exile out with a whip of thongs. Reference to the temple, in the figurative language of the Bible and New Testament, always symbolizes the human organism. "Know ye not that your bodies are the Temple of the living God?" Solomon's temple is an allegory of the physical body of man and woman. Soul – of man's temple – the house, church, Beth or temple made without sound of "saw or hammer."

Hate, envy criticism, jealousy, competition, selfishness, war, suicide and murder are largely caused by acid conditions of the blood, producing changes by chemical poison and irritation of the brain cells, the keys upon which soul plays "Divine harmonies" or plays "fantastic tricks before high heaven," according to the arrangement of chemical molecules in the wondrous laboratory of the soul. Without a proper balance of the alkaline salt, the agent of peace and love, man is fit for "treason, stratagem and spoils."

*This complete introductory section is adapted from:
The Chemistry and Wonders of the Human Body by Dr. George Carey.

The chemistry of life points to the reason why man is unbalanced. Poise of tissue, nerve fluid, blood and brains cells, as well as muscular fiber, are conditions precedent to mental or soul poise. A man thinks and acts according to the organism in or through which the ego operates.

The basis of the human body are twelve minerals, lime (calcium), iron, potash, silica, sodium, magnesia, etc, etc. They are found in the ashes of the cremated body, or, in reality constitute the ashes. Before man ceases to be sick, before envy, strife, hatred, competition, selfishness, war, and murder cease on Earth, man must build his body on a plan that will express mind on the plane of altruism and love. The perfectly balanced body will enable the mind to cognize oneness of being. From this concept comes peace on Earth, and good will between man and man.

The knowledge of life chemistry will bring man to his Divine estate in the kingdom of harmony and love. This kingdom is forming in the chemicalizing mass of God's creative compounds. Out from the chemistry of elements, principles, monads and molecules; out of oxygen, hydrogen, nitrogen, carbon, helium, uranium, radium, aurium, argentum, sodium, potassium and iron – out from molecules composing the body of universal energy – a man and woman will be born (real sons of God) who will bear away the sins of the world.

MATERIA MEDICA FOR NAT PHOS

Adapted from: *The Biochemic System of Medicine, Materia Medica* by Dr. George Carey

The fluids of the body contain both alkali and acid; but a deficiency in acid never occurs, because it is organic, and, like protein, is always present in sufficient quantities when proper food is taken. As it is necessary, absolutely necessary, that a proper balance of calcium phosphate molecules be present to work with protein and properly distribute it and incorporate it into bone and other tissue, so it is absolutely necessary that a proper amount of the phosphate of soda be present as a worker with acid, to combine with it and thus form new compounds. Thus it will be seen that "an excess of acid" is a misnomer, and that the true way to put it is: "A deficiency exists in the phosphate of sodium." (Nat Phos) And here again comes in the creative power inherent in the inorganic salts.

Organic matter has no creative power, no more than has brick. The brick mason, given a supply of brick, possesses the power to create the brick wall.

The inorganic mineral salts have the power to create, when furnished with the proper material. But the material is always present; it is the laborers that are scarce in disease. The only trouble that ever arises is a deficiency in workmen. A lack of proper balance of the alkaline cell salt in gastric juice will allow ferments to arise and so retard digestion that the lining quickly becomes involved. An inspissation (thickening) of bile occurs, and bilious diarrhea or other bilious disorders follow. For such conditions Nat Sulph must be given also, although Nat Phos would have prevented such results.

Characteristic Indications

(Note: The remedies in parentheses are support for Nat Phos.)

Head – Headache on the crown of head or in the forehead, with feeling as if the skull were too full. Sick headache, with vomiting of sour fluids (alternate Ferrum Phos). Headache on awakening in the morning. **Note color of the tongue; if there is a creamy deposit on the back part, this salt is indicated.** Very severe headaches on top of the head, with intense pressure and heat (Ferrum Phos). Some gastric troubles usually exist and should be relieved. Headaches, with pain in the stomach and ejection of frothy, sour fluid. Giddiness, when gastric derangements are present (alternate Ferrum Phos).

Eyes – Inflammation of eyes, **when secreting a golden-yellow creamy matter.** Eyes glued together in the morning with a creamy discharge. Any disease of the eyes, when accompanied with the characteristic creamy discharge (note also color of root of tongue and palate). **Squinting**, when caused by irritation **from worms**, to remove the cause (Mag Phos).

Ears – One ear red, hot and frequently itchy, accompanied by gastric derangement and acidity. Outer ears sore and scabby, with creamy discharge, or the scabs have a creamy, yellow appearance (not color of tongue). Heat and burning of the ears, with gastric symptoms (Ferrum Phos).

Nose – Picking at the nose, generally a symptom of worms or of an acid condition **of the stomach. Cold in the head, with yellow, creamy discharge from the nose; itching of the nose**, with acidity. **Note color of tongue, palate and roof of mouth.**

Face – Face red and blotched, without fever; blotches come and go suddenly; white about the mouth and nose, indicating worms or acid condition of the stomach, associated with **creamy colored tongue** and sour, acid rising.

Mouth – Creamy, yellow coating at the back part of the roof of mouth. Creamy, golden-yellow exudation from tonsils and pharynx. **Sour, acid taste in the mouth** sometimes accompanied with canker sores (Kali Mur, Kali Phos).

Teeth – Children grind their teeth during sleeping, associated with gastric derangements or worms. **Gastric derangements during teething.**

Tongue – "The great keynote for this remedy is the moist creamy or golden-yellow coating at the back part of the tongue" (Drs. Boericke and Dewey).

Throat – Sore, raw feeling in the throat; tonsils and throat inflamed, with creamy, yellow, moist coating. Catarrh of the throat; tonsils covered with the characteristic discharge of this salt, usually associated with acid condition of the stomach. **False diphtheria, with creamy coating of the palate** and back part of the tongue.

Gastric symptoms – All conditions of the stomach where there are sour, acid risings or the tongue has a moist, creamy yellow coating. Dyspepsia, with acid risings (alternate with Ferrum Phos, to strengthen digestion). Gastric abrasions, superficial ulcerations, pain after eating, calls for this remedy if the accompanying acid conditions are present (Calc Phos, Ferrum Phos). Gastric derangements causing flatulence, headache, and giddiness. **Morning sickness, with vomiting of sour fluids.** Nausea, with sour risings. Stomachache from the presence of worms or acidity of the stomach. Ulceration of the stomach, when the **least amount of food causes pain** and tongue and palate have the characteristic creamy, yellow coating. Ulceration of the stomach, with vomiting of sour, acid fluids or substance like coffee grounds; follow with Ferrum Phos and Calc Phos. Vomiting sour, acid fluids (not food). Infants vomit curdled milk.

Abdomen and stool – Diarrhea, especially of children, with green, sour smelling stools, caused by an acid condition. Flatulent colic, with green, sour smelling stools or vomiting of curdled masses. **Diarrhea**, when there is **much straining at stool or constant urging to stool**, with passing of jelly-like masses of mucus, indicating acidity (Kali Mur). Worms of all kinds, with accompanying symptoms of picking the nose, itching of the anus, pain in the abdomen, acidity of the stomach, restless sleep, etc. (Injections of same remedy). Ulceration of the bowels, when characteristic symptoms are present (Ferrum Phos).

Urinary organs – Frequent urination, with **inability to retain urine**, with corresponding symptoms of acidity; more frequently seen in children (Ferrum Phos). Dark red urine, with rheumatism (Ferrum Phos).

Male sexual organs – Seminal emissions, without dreams, or when followed by weakness and trembling. Irregularity of sexual desires, whether gone or increased, when there are other indications of acid condition of the system.

Female sexual organs – All secretions from uterus or vagina which are acid, creamy, yellow and watery. **Sterility caused by acid secretions** from the vagina, proving fatal to the spermatozoa. Leucorrhea, with watery, creamy, yellow, acid discharge, causing itching, rawness and soreness of the parts. Discharges smell sour and sickening. Irregularity of monthly periods, when accompanied with acid leucorrhea and frontal headache; also vomiting of acid fluids (not food).

Pregnancy – Morning sickness of pregnancy, with sour, acid vomit (not food), or other acid conditions. Nausea, with sour risings.

Respiratory organs – In consumption (tuberculosis), when the expectoration causes soreness of the lips or rawness of the tongue and mouth.

Circulatory organs – Palpitation and irregularity of heart's action, caused from imperfect digestion. **Trembling about the heart; always worse after eating.** The diet and bowels should be looked at carefully.

Back and extremities – In all cases of acute or chronic articular rheumatism this remedy is indicated and should be prescribed alternately or inter-currently with other remedies. Nat Phos is a remedy for the acid diathesis (tendency), which many believe is (if not the sole cause) at least a formidable attendant upon this distressing diseases. **Rheumatic pains in the joints,** weak feeling in the legs. Acid, sour-smelling perspiration. Cracking and creaking of joints, with pain and soreness. Gout (Nat Sulph).

Nervous symptoms – Squinting and grinding of teeth, with intestinal irritation from worms. Nervousness, with trembling and palpitation of the heart, from acid condition of the stomach.

Skin – Eczema of the skin, when accompanied **with acrid, creamy, yellow secretions.** Chafing of the skin, with soreness and rawness in little children; **note characteristic symptoms** of this salt (Nat Mur). Erythema, "rose rash" (alternate with Ferrum Phos). Crusta lactea (condition afflicting infants and little children that creates scaly crusts on the scalp). Pimples all over the body, like flea bites, with itching and acid symptoms. Hives.

Tissues – Discharges from any mucus membrane or sore in the flesh, of a creamy, yellow or honey color, which can be traced to a disturbance of the molecules of sodium phosphate, is said to favor the deposit of Calc Phos in bone diseases. Rheumatism, with acid symptoms.

Febrile conditions – Acid, **sour-smelling perspiration** during any disease. Fever, with vomiting of sour fluids. Acid symptoms during the course of any febrile disease. Flashes of heat from indigestion, often causing frontal headache.

Sleep – Restless sleep from worm troubles, gritting the teeth and screaming in sleep, with itching of anus and picking of nose.

FACIAL SIGNS OF NAT PHOS DEFICIENCY

Yellow. The face has yellowish, sunken, or bloated skin. There are yellow points in the corners of the eyes and show an inability to metabolize fat (high cholesterol). Yellow points in mouth corners show liver involvement.

There is a **fatty appearance** that is shiny (the pores appear open, especially on nose, forehead, and chin). We can also see a greasy cheese-like appearance on the skin. Sweating on the face can contribute to blackhead development.

Blackheads are often seen in Nat Phos deficiencies. Small black pores are mostly seen on the nose, corners of the mouth, forehead and

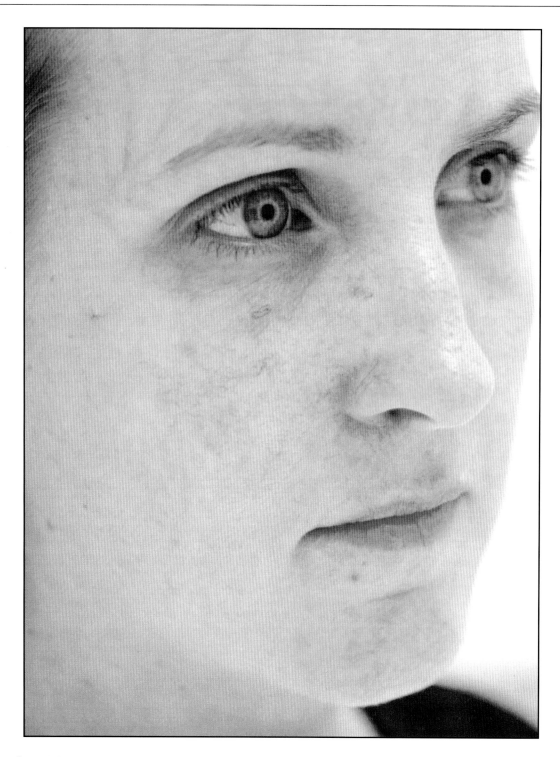

Nat Phos (a)

This woman's chin is red with acne, characteristic of a severe Nat Phos deficiency. The tip of her nose is shiny and the skin is translucent above her right eye, which shows a Silicea deficiency. The brownish circles under the eyes are a sign of a Calc Fluor deficiency. The redness of the cheeks are an indication of Kali Mur deficiency.

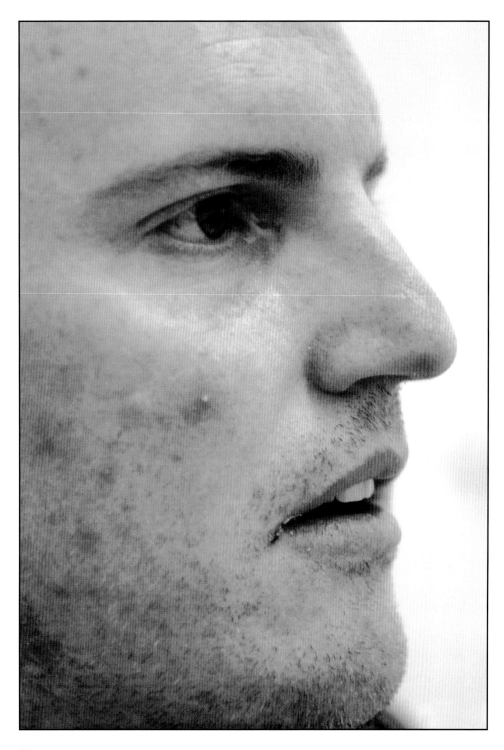

Nat Phos (b)

The pimples on the right side of this man's face show a Nat Phos deficiency. He also has the bluish-black circle under the eye of a Ferrum Phos deficiency. There is a red forehead from a Mag Phos deficiency, and the shine of the forehead is a Silicea deficiency symptom.

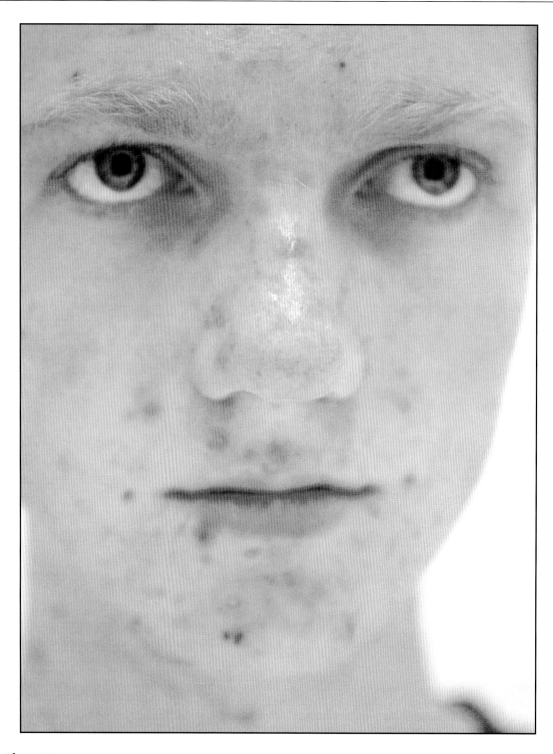

Nat Phos (c)

This photo highlights the typical red acne of Nat Phos. There is also a deficiency of Silicea noted by the deep-set eyes. His dark brownish-black circles show a Calc Fluor deficiency. The nose has large pores, indicative of a Nat Mur deficiency.

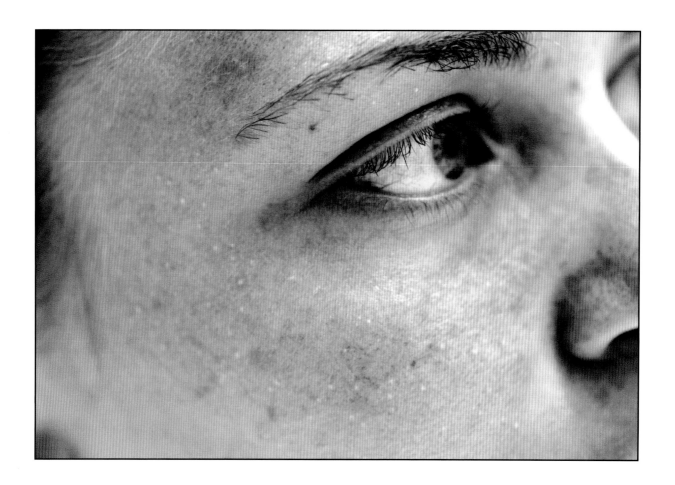

Nat Phos (d)

This woman has the redness of a Nat Phos deficiency and acne signs. The small yellow pimples are a Calc Sulph deficiency. She has dark bluish-black circles under her eye – a Ferrum Phos deficiency sign.

chin, pimples, acne. Most white discharges are a symptom of kidney damage.

Hanging cheeks, hamster appearance, double chin.

Red nose (Dyspepsia, poor digestion) are combined with spotty skin; also, red skin after eating shows a Nat Phos deficiency.

THERAPEUTIC INDEX FOR NAT PHOS

Adapted from *Therapeutic Index* (1890) by Dr. W. H. Schuessler

Acidity.

Diabetes mellitus, if acidity predominates, etc. (Nat Sulph)

Nat Phos Summary

ORGAN AND TISSUE AFFINITIES
Mucus membranes, lower stomach, bile ducts, nerves, stomach, intestines, lymphatics.

MODALITIES
Symptoms worse < milk, sugar, mental activity, during menses, thunderstorms, sex.
Symptoms better > pressure, cold, and open air.

DEFICIENCY SYMPTOMS
Heartburn, acne, digestion, hypoglycemia, blackheads, swollen glands, sugar cravings, sour smell, acidity conditions, candida.

DISEASE CONDITIONS
Parasites, creamy yellow discharges, acidity, jaundice, candida, acne, blackheads.

Diarrhea, caused by excess of acids, sour smelling.

Eyes, discharge of yellow, creamy matter.

Gastric derangements, with predominating acidity.

Intermittent fever, sour taste, vomiting of acid, sour masses.

Morning sickness, with vomiting of sour masses.

Scabs, if golden yellow, like honey.

Secretions, discharges of slime or mucus, if green.

Secretions, discharges of matter, if green, also if acidity exist.

Tongue, coating at the back, golden yellow, creamy.

Vomiting of acid (sour) masses.

Worms, intestinal, with characteristic symptoms.

ASTROLOGY OF NAT PHOS
Libra: The Loins of the Zodiac
September 23 to October 23

Adapted from: *Cell Salts of Salvation* by Dr. George Carey

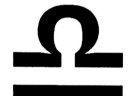

The Sun enters the domain of Libra on September 23 and remains there until October 23. "Libra" is a Latin word meaning scales or balance. Sodium, or natrum phosphate (Nat Phos), holds the balance between acids and normal fluids of the human body. This alkaline cell salt is made from bone ash or by neutralizing orthophosphoric acid with carbonate of sodium. A certain amount of acid is necessary, and is always present in the blood, nerves, stomach and liver fluids. The apparent excess of acid is nearly always due to a deficiency in the alkaline, Libra, salt.

The people of the world never needed the alkaline or Libra salt more than they do at the present time, while wars and rumors of wars strut upon the "stage of life" (1918).

The governing planet of this air sign is Venus. The gems associated with Libra are diamond and opal, and the colors are black, crimson and light blue. In Bible alchemy, Libra represents Reuben, the first son of Jacob. Reuben means "vision of the Sun." In the symbolism of the New Testament, Libra corresponds with the disciple Peter. Peter is derived from "petra," a stone or mineral. "On thee, Peter (mineral), will I build my church," viz., beth, house, body or temple.

CHAPTER 13

Nat Sulph

This salt may be obtained by the action of sulphuric acid on sodium chloride (common salt). This cell salt is found in the intercellular fluids, liver and pancreas. Its principal work is to regulate the supply of water in the human organism.*

The blood becomes overcharged with water, either from the oxidation of organic matter or from inhaling air that contains more aqueous vapor than is required to produce normal blood. This condition of air is liable to prevail whenever the temperature is above 70 degrees.

One molecule of Nat Sulph (also referred to as natrum sulphate, sulphate of sodium or Glauber's Salts) has the power, chemical intelligence, to take up and carry away two molecules, or twice its bulk, of water. The blood does not become overcharged with water from water taken into the stomach, but from the water lifted by expansion caused by heat above 70 degrees and held in the air and thus breathed into the arteries through the lungs. Based on the above, we see that there is more work for this salt in hot weather than during cold weather. So-called "malaria," Latin for "bad air," is due to a lack of this tissue salt. Water, lifted from swamps or clear streams or lakes by the action of the sun's heat, is the same, for heat does not evaporate and lift poisonous, disintegrating organic matter from a swamp or marsh, but the water only.

Therefore, it is not some impurity in the air that causes chills, etc., but an oversupply of water which thins the bile and distributes it through the organism. Nature's effort to get rid of the surplus water by nervous, muscular and vascular contraction, on the principle of wringing water from a cloth, causes the spasm called "chills." Proof of this theory is found in the fact that perspiration follows the chill. It generally requires about 48 hours to again over-charge the blood and bring on another chill.

*This complete introductory section is adapted from:
The Chemistry and Wonders of the Human Body by Dr. George Carey.

Cold, dry air always cures chill, and be it known that all cold air is dry air. The cure for chills when cold air cannot be had is Nat Sulph in biochemic potency. Yellow fever is caused by too much water in bile and other liver fluids. These fluids are distributed through the system, and in their union with oil, protein, etc., become vitiated (corrupted) and cause the yellow skin.

Nat Sulph in crude form is known as Glauber's Salts, and is too course to be taken up by the mucus membrane absorbents and carried into the circulation; it must be triturated with sugar of milk, according to the biochemic method, up to the third or sixth decimal before using a remedy to supply the blood. Glauber's Salts, crude sodium sulphate, acts as a cathartic, and cathartics are never used in the biochemic system of healing.

When man learns to keep his blood at the proper rate of motion by the proper dynamos – the mineral salts – he will not fear fevers, microbes, mosquitoes, nor devils.

MATERIA MEDICA FOR NAT SULPH

Adapted from: *The Biochemic System of Medicine, Materia Medica* by Dr. George Carey

This inorganic salt is found in the intercellular fluids and its principal office is to regulate the water in the tissue, blood and fluids of the body. A deficiency of this salt prevents the elimination of such water from the tissue as is produced by oxidation of organic matter, while Nat Mur properly distributes the water in tissue, as has been shown. Nat Sulph regulates the amount by having the power to eliminate any excess that may, from any cause, be present. First, decomposition of lactic acid with Nat Phos leaves a residue of water to be gotten rid of, and sodium sulphate must be present in proper quantity, or a hydrogenoid (water-logged) condition will arise. Second, in hot weather, where water is present, it is held in solution by the heat of the sun in the

atmospheric air, and thus enters the blood through the lungs. Those who are weakly, whose digestion is in any way impaired, are then liable to malarial troubles, because the circulation is not able to eliminate the excess of water from the blood because of a lack of proper quantity of Nat Sulph molecules to do the work. To speak from a chemical view, one molecule of Nat Sulph has the power to take up and carry out of the organism two molecules of water.

Biochemistry has established the fact that chills and fever (or ague), cholera, yellow fever and all ailments incident to hot weather, are basically caused by an excess of water in the blood, and probably in intercellular fluids; and that all such conditions arise from the inability of the digestion and assimilation to furnish sufficient quantity of Nat Sulph to carry off the excess of water breathed into the blood through the lungs. Let us take a case of malaria. Hot weather causes a rapid evaporation of water, especially in low, marshy districts, and regions where there are many ponds and other small bodies of water. This water is held in solution in the atmosphere, and is, of course, taken into the blood through the lungs by the act of breathing; thus the blood becomes overcharged with water.

The cell salt Nat Sulph has an affinity for oxygen, and oxygen has an affinity for water, and thus, in health, Nat Sulph is able to eliminate this excess of water from the system. If however, from any cause, a deficiency of Nat Sulph exists in the system, this surplus water cannot be carried off. Thus a suitable breeding place in the blood is supplied for the plasmodium malariac or haematozoa of Laveran (maleria), a vegetable microorganism to which the active manifestations of malarial fever are due. The plasmodium is introduced into the human system by a species of mosquito, the anopheles, which carries the organism in its blood, and transmits it through its bites.

When once established in the blood, the plasmodium causes a series of paroxysms (spasms), nearly always occurring with remarkable regularity, either at the end of 24, 48, or 72 hours. If occurring at the expiration of 24 hours from the beginning of the proceeding paroxysms, the fever is said to be of *the quotidian type*. If the interval between paroxysms is 48 hours, the paroxysms occurring every third day, the fever is of *the tertian type*. If the interval is 72 hours, the paroxysm recurring on the fourth day, it is *a quartan fever*. The quotidian and tertian types of intermittent fever are the most common, the quartan being comparatively rare.

There is also a form of malarial fever known as "remittent fever," in which the temperature varies, but never gets as low as normal. This fever ranges from mild to severe, and lasts from one to two weeks. Quinine seems to possess a specific action against the plasmodium malaria, but as its maximum effect is not obtained from 4-6 hours after its administration, in the quotidian type it should be given 8 hours before the expected chill, and repeated; in the tertian, 12 hours before, and repeated; in the quartan type, 15 hours before the expected chill, and repeated. Then, also, 15-grain doses are usually sufficient in the milder types, while in the more sever types 30 to 60 grains are often required. The quinine should be given in powder as soft capsules easily dissolved.

Quinine is not, however, the only or the most important remedy in malarial fever. The basic cause of the trouble is an excess of water in the blood, which has provided a suitable breeding place for the plasmodium malaria, and this excess of water must be removed, so that a recurrence of the disease may be prevented, and a permanent restoration to health assured. This excess of water is due to a deficiency of the cell salt Nat Sulph, and it is only by supplying this lacking salt that the condition can be overcome. Nat Sulph is thus the chief remedy in malarial fevers. When the trouble has continued for some time, the nervous system is frequently affected by a lack of Kali Phos, and this salt is also needed. The fever, too,

always calls for Ferrum Phos.

So, we find that among the inorganic salts in the human economy that Nat Sulph works with water, keeps bile and pancreatic juice at normal consistency, regulates the supply of water in intercellular fluid, and eliminates the excess of water from the blood.

Characteristic Indications

(Note: The remedies in parentheses are support for Nat Sulph.)

Mental symptoms – Irritation due to biliousness (excess of bile); tendency to suicide, with wildness and irritability, from an excessive secretion of bile. **Feels discouraged and despondent**; worse in the morning and in damp weather.

Head – Headache on top of head; very severe, burning and throbbing (note color of tongue). Sick headache, with bitter taste in the mouth, vomiting of bile or bilious diarrhea. **Headache, with dizziness** or drowsiness; often the precursor of jaundice. Vertigo, giddiness from excessive secretion of bile; **tongue has a dirty, greenish-gray or greenish-brown coating** at the back part; bitter taste in the mouth. Violent pains to head; spasmodic symptoms and delirium (Ferrum Phos, Mag Phos).

Eyes – Yellowness of the conjunctiva. **Burning of the edges of the lids**, with lachrymation (tears). Chronic conjunctivitis, with large blister-like granulations of the lids.

Ears – Earache, lightning-like pain through the ears; worse in damp weather.

Nose – Ozeana syphilitica (bad smell of nose from tissue destruction), worse in damp, wet weather. Nasal catarrh (congestion). Dryness and burning in the nose. Pus changes to green when exposed to light.

Face – Yellow, sallow or jaundiced face, due to biliousness. (Note appearance of tongue.) **Erysipelas** (redness) of the face, **smooth, red, shiny swelling** (for the fever, Ferrum Phos).

Mouth – Bad taste in the mouth, always full of slime, thick and tenacious, greenish-white. Bitter taste in mouth. Constant hawking of foul, slimy mucus from the trachea, esophagus and stomach.

Tongue – Dirty, greenish-gray or greenish-brown coating on the root (back) of the tongue, with slime. Bitter taste in the mouth.

Throat – When vomiting of green water occurs in diphtheria, this remedy should be given intercurrently with chief remedy (Kali Mur). Throat sore, with feeling of a lump when swallowing. Catarrh of the pharynx and throat, with thick, tenacious, grayish mucus, if tongue symptoms correspond.

Gastric symptoms – Biliousness, caused from the liver secreting an excess of bile. The tongue should be noted carefully; a greenish-gray or greenish-brown coating indicates an excess of bile, while a white or gray coating denotes a deficiency of bile, and requires Kali Mur. Bitter taste in mouth. Mouth full of slime. Bilious colic, with bitter taste in mouth (see tongue symptoms). Lead (poisoning) colic (very frequent doses and low triturations). Vomiting of bile, with bitter taste, dizziness and headache. Vomiting of greenish water, tasting bitter. Jaundice from vexation, oversecretion of bile, with coated tongue; bilious, green evacuations; yellow eyeballs or sallow skin. Sick headache from gastric derangement (note tongue). Cutting pains in region of liver. Enlargement of liver; worse lying on the left side. Irritable liver (Kali Phos). Pain in left hypochondriac region (upper abdomen), frequently accompanied by a cough.

Abdomen and stool – Diarrhea, with dark, greenish, bilious stools, or vomiting of bile (note coating of tongue). Loose morning stool; worse in cold, wet weather. Heat in the lower bowels and rectum, accompanied by bilious evacuations. Flatulent colic, irritable liver, frequently after a mental strain (Kali Phos). Liver sensitive, sore to touch, with sharp, shooting pains. Congestion of liver (Ferrum Phos). Cutting pains in abdomen (Mag Phos, Ferrum Phos). Typhlitis, to aid in reducing the inflammation (in alternation with Ferrum Phos, the chief remedy). Looseness of bowels in old people. All symptoms worse, or after a spell of, wet weather.

Urinary organs – Diabetes, chief remedy, for the sugar and general waste from the kidneys. Lithic (stone) deposit in urine; looks brick-dust and clings to the side of the vessel. Gravel (stones), with gouty symptoms, in bilious persons, excessive secretion of urine, when diabetic. Sandy deposit in the urine (note color of tongue).

Male sexual organs – Hydrocele (swollen scrotum) (Calc Phos). Preputial edema (prepuce of penis swollen) (Nat Mur in alternation). Chronic syphilis, when corresponding symptoms are present. Condyloma (wart-like growth) of syphilitic origin, internally and externally. Chronic gonorrhea, with characteristic discharge.

Female sexual organs – Profuse menses, with morning diarrhea, or colic and constipation. Note color of tongue and other characteristic symptoms

Pregnancy – Morning sickness, with vomiting of bilious fluids, bitter taste in the mouth.

Respiratory organs – Asthma, violent attacks, with greenish, purulent expectoration; very copious. Asthma, worse in damp, wet weather, with loose evacuations in the morning. Bronchial catarrh, harsh breathing. All symptoms worse in damp, rainy weather. Observe coating on root of tongue and color of expectoration.

Circulatory organs – Vertigo, with giddiness: feeling of pressure and uneasiness in region of heart.

Back and extremities – Rheumatism, for the bilious symptoms, when present; intercurrently or in alternation with the chief remedy. Gout, acute or chronic cases (Ferrum Phos). Spinal meningitis, for the drawing back of the neck, spasm in the back, and violent determination of the blood to the head; violent pains in the neck and back of head. Arthritis, acute; patient should abstain from intoxicating liquors

Nervous symptoms – Lassitude (tiredness); tired and weary feelings when accompanied by bilious symptoms, jaundiced skin, yellow eyeballs, etc. **Hands and feet twitch during sleep.**

Skin – All diseases of the skin, with exudation of yellowish water; generally accompanied by other bilious symptoms. Inflammations of the skin, with yellow, watery exudation. Skin affections, with vesicular eruptions (blisters) containing yellowish water; **moist yellowish scales on the skin, with bilious symptoms.** Chafed skin of infants (Nat Mur, Nat Phos). Pemphigus water vesicles (crops of blisters) all over the body containing yellowish, watery secretions. Eczema, with watery exudations and bilious symptoms. Erysipelas ("rose"), smooth, red, shiny, tingly, or painful swelling of the skin (alternate with Ferrum Phos: note condition of tongue). Fistulous abscess (boil-like) of long standing. Discharging of watery pus, surrounded by a broad bluish border.

Tissues – Dropsy (swelling) invading the areolar (brown border) tissues of the body. Infiltration. Yellowish, watery secretions from any tissue. Smooth, edematous swellings. **Consumption** (tuberculosis), when the **expectoration is yellow, watery, and green**; also when corresponding bilious symptoms exist.

Febrile conditions – **Intermittent fever (ague)**; this is the **chief remedy** in all its stages. Vomiting of bile, also brown or black fluids, with bitter taste. Bilious fever. Yellow fever, if it assumes the severe, bilious, remittent fever form, with greenish-yellow, brown, or black vomit (alternate Ferrum Phos, for the fever). Observe carefully the **characteristic** dirty greenish-gray or greenish-brown **coating of the tongue** in all febrile conditions.

Sleep – Drowsiness and weariness with bilious symptoms, frequently preceding attacks of jaundice (note coating of tongue). Dull, sleepy, and stupid in the morning; better in the evening. Much dreaming, with **heavy, anxious dreams**, attacks of "nightmare," with bilious symptoms (Nat Mur, Kali Phos).

Modalities – All symptoms are worse in the morning and in damp, wet weather; feels better in dry, warm atmosphere. Complaints from living in damp buildings, basements, etc., or from eating water-plants, fish, etc. **Symptoms aggravated** by the use of **water** in any form. Conditions which tend to increase the water in the system, such as living in low, marshy places,

---

Nat Sulph Summary

ORGAN AND TISSUE AFFINITIES
Liver, gallbladder, pancreas, colon, head.

MODALITIES
Symptoms worse < cold damp weather, head injuries, lying on the left side, light, music, veggies, cold food and drink.
Symptoms better > open air, passing gas, warmth, pressure, breakfast, sitting up.

DEFICIENCY SYMPTOMS
Swollen hands and feet, depression, suicidal feelings, bad gas, itching skin, skin has a greenish tinge, lower eyelid sacks.

DISEASE CONDITIONS
Head injuries, bad gas, epilepsy after head injury, spinal meningitis, diabetes, photophobia, asthma especially in children, bitter taste, yellowish discharges.

"ague districts," will cause a molecular disturbance of Nat Sulf.

FACIAL SIGNS OF NAT SULPH DEFICIENCY

Greenish-yellow coloring of the skin is the second color that is connected with yellow. The brownish yellow coloring is the Kali Sulf deficiency sign. It appears as a greenish yellow or a yellowish green. The more greenish is often the sign of Nat Sulf deficiency. As with Kali Sulf, this coloring is most often seen on the chin. This coloring is often seen above the eyes and can be seen as an "A" form from the root of the nose. It is also seen around the corners of the eyes. It may also be seen as a shimmering color on the cheeks.

Green to grass-green coloring is the color of a person before they vomit, especially around the chin. This shows that the liver is overwhelmed and shows a Nat Sulf deficiency. This is often seen in an acute situation.

Bluish-red coloring is the second Nat Sulf deficiency color. This is most often seen on the top of the nose, but can occur on the entire face. This is often seen when the liver is overtaxed. This appears to be an inflammatory condition, because the blood is overburdened with toxins. (Ferrum Phos, inflammation is more acute.)

The **"alcohol nose"** is dark red and is a chronic condition. The alcoholic has a huge Natrum Sulf deficiency from liver toxicity. This is seen in a bluish-red coloring.

Not only do we see the **swollen eye sacks** directly under the eyes, but these can extend to the borders of the cheeks. This is often seen as a kidney weakness but often involves the liver. It is often treated with Nat Mur for the kidneys, but if it fails, look to the liver and Nat Sulf. The swollen sacks may be a sign of body toxicity that the liver can't remove without sufficient supplies of Nat Sulf.

Smelly gas is not a facial analysis but an important sign nonetheless. Large doses of Nat Sulf usually can help in a few days.

THERAPEUTIC INDEX FOR NAT SULPH

Adapted from: *Therapeutic Index* (1890) by Dr. W. H. Schuessler

Diarrhea, bilious, green bile.
Erysipelas "rose," smooth, shiny. (Rosy skin problem)
Gastric derangement, (indigestion) with bitter taste.
Intermittent fever, with vomiting of bile, tongue greenish yellow with or without bitter taste.
Polyuria simplex, excessive secretion of urine.
Preputial edema (swelling penis head)
Scrotal edema (swelling of testicles)
Secretions, with or without vesicles, which are watery not sticky.
Skin, edematous inflammation (swelling inflammations of skin).
Tongue, dirty, brownish-greenish coating, generally with bitter taste.
Vomiting of pure bile, bilious; including morning sickness, bitter taste.

ASTROLOGY OF NAT SULPH
Taurus: The Winged Bull of the Zodiac
April 19 to May 20

Adapted from *Cell Salts of Salvation* by Dr. George Carey

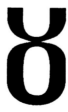 The ancients were not "primitive men." There never was a first man, or a primitive man. Man is an eternal verity – the Truth – and Truth never had a beginning.

The Winged Bull of Nineveh is a symbol of the great truth that substance is materialized air, and that all so-called solid substances may be

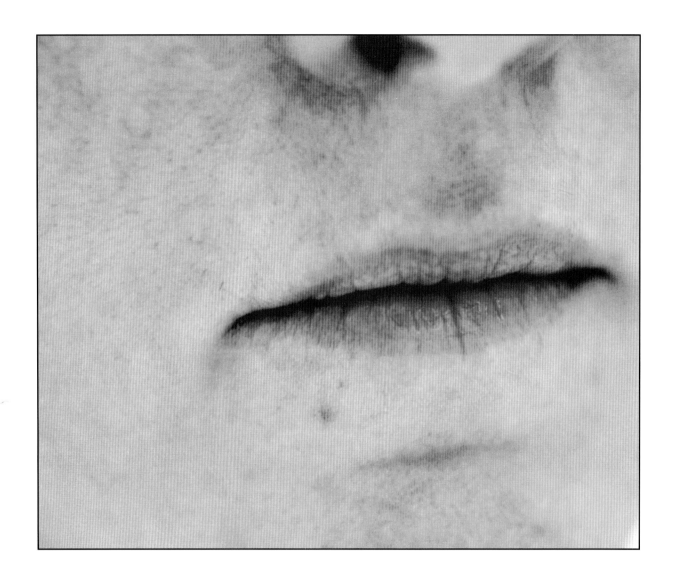

Nat Sulph (a)

The greenish cast around this subject's mouth points to a Nat Sulph deficiency. The reddish chin is a sign of Nat Phos deficiency. The large pores are a Nat Mur deficiency sign.

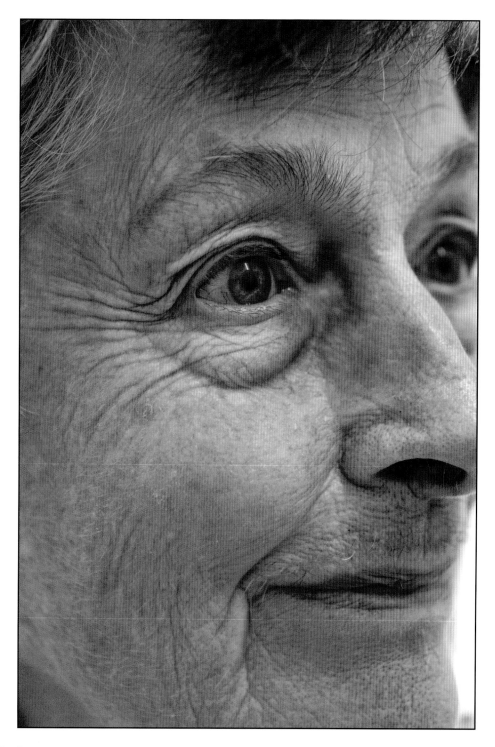

Nat Sulph (b)

This woman's eyes have large eye bags representative of a severe Nat Sulph deficiency. The crow's-feet at the edge of the eyes are a Calc Fluor deficiency. The wrinkles all around show a Silicea deficiency.

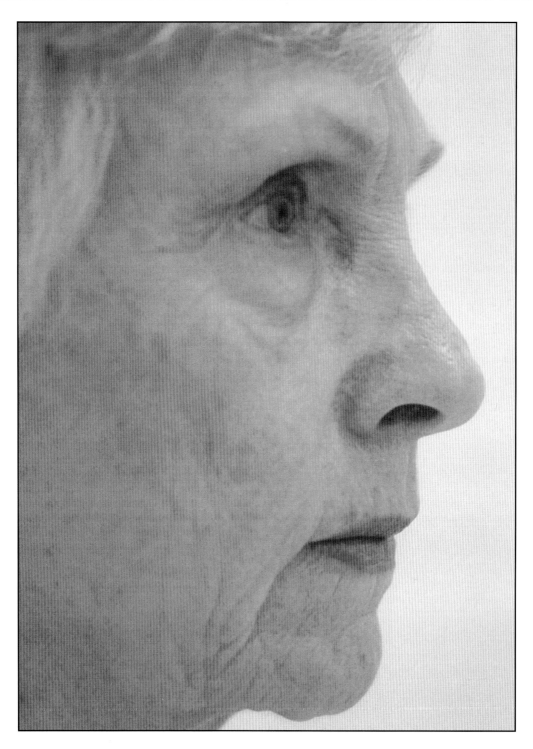

Nat Sulph (c)

This woman has large eye bags, a sign of Nat Sulph deficiency. The redness of the nose is also a Nat Sulph deficiency sign. The wrinkles show a Silicea deficiency. She also has dark bluish-black circles under the eyes, which are a Ferrum Phos deficiency.

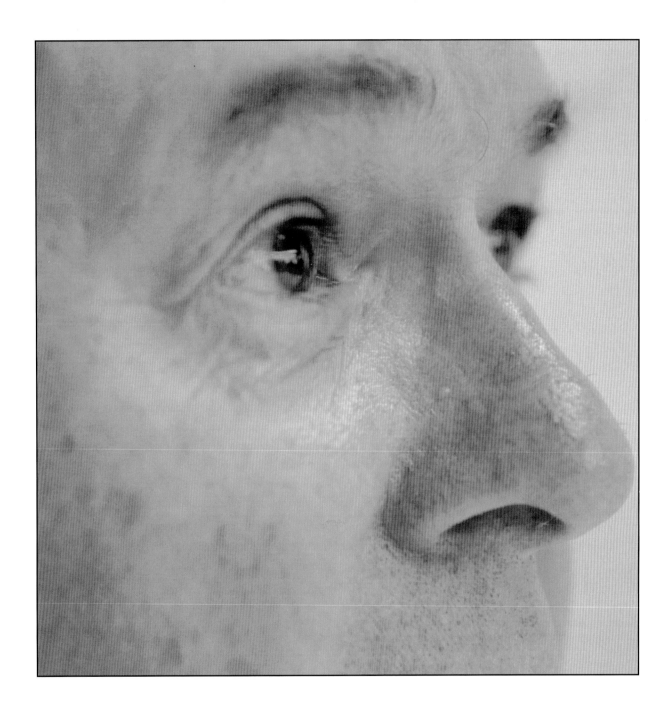

Nat Sulph (d)

The color of this man's nose is the chronic dark red of a Nat Sulph deficiency. He has large pores on his nose, a Nat Mur deficiency. The brownish-black circle under the eye indicates a Calc Fluor deficiency. He has a few brown spots showing a slight Kali Sulph deficiency.

resolved into air. Taurus is an earth sign, but earth is precipitated air elements. This chemical fact was known to the scientists of the Taurian age (over 4,000 years ago); therefore they carved the emblem of their zodiacal sign with wings.

Those borne between the dates April 19th and May 20th, can descend very deep into materiality or soar "High as the Heaven where Taurus wheels," as written by Edwin Markham, who is a Taurus native. What can be finer than the following from this noted Taurian, he who has sprouted the wings of spiritual concept:

It is a vision waiting and aware, and you must bring it down, oh men of worth, bring down the New Republic hung in air. And make for it foundations on the Earth.

Air is the "raw material" for blood, and when it is drawn in, or breathed in, rather, by the "infinite alchemist," to the blood vessels, it unites with the philosopher's stone, mineral salts, and in the human laboratory creates blood.

So, then, blood is the elixir of life, the "Ichor of the Gods." Nat Sulph chemically corresponds to the physical and mental characteristics of those born in the Taurus month. Taurus is represented by the cerebellum, or lower brain, and neck.

A deficiency in Nat Sulph in the blood is always manifested by pains in the back of the head, sometimes extending down the spine, and then affecting the liver. The first cell salt to become deficient in symptoms of disease in the Taurus native is Nat Sulph.

The chief office of Nat Sulph is to eliminate the excess of water from the body. In hot weather the atmosphere becomes heavily laden with water and is thus breathed into the blood through the lungs. One molecule of the Taurus salt has the chemical power to take up and carry out of the system two molecules of water.

Blood does not become overcharged with water from the water we drink, but from the atmosphere overcharged with aqueous vapor drawn from water in rivers, lakes or swamps, by heat of the sun above 70 degrees in shade. The more surplus water there is to be thrown out of blood the more Nat Sulph is required.

All so-called bilious or malarial troubles are simply a chemical effect or action caused by deficiency of Nat Sulph.

Chills and fever are nature's method of getting rid of surplus water by squeezing it out of the blood through violent muscular, nervous and vascular spasms. No "shakes" or ague can occur if blood were properly balanced chemically.

The governing planet of Taurus is Venus. Its gems are moss-agate and emerald, and its astral colors are red and lemon yellow. In Bible alchemy, Taurus represents Asher, the eighth son of Jacob, and means "blessedness" or "happiness." In the symbolism of the New Testament, Taurus corresponds with the disciple Thaddeus, meaning "firmness," or "led by love."

CHAPTER 14

Silicea

Silicea (or silica) is made by fusing crude silica with carbonate of soda: dissolve the residue, filter, and precipitate by hydrochloric acid.*

This salt is the surgeon of the human organism. Silica is found in the hair, skin, nails, periosteum (the membrane covering and protecting the bone), the nerve sheath, called "neurilemma," and a trace is found in bone tissue. The surgical qualities of silica lie in the fact that its particles are sharp cornered. A piece of quartz is a sample of the finer particles. Reduce silica to an impalpable powder and the microscope reveals the fact that the molecules are still pointed and jagged like a large piece of quartz rock. In all cases, where it becomes necessary that decaying organic matter be discharged from any part of the body by the process of suppuration (pus), these sharp-pointed particles are pushed forward by the marvelous intelligence that operates without ceasing, day and night, in the wondrous human body, and, like a lancet, cuts a passage to the surface for the discharge of the pus. Nowhere in all the records of physiology or biological research can anything be found more wonderful than the chemical and mechanical operation of this Divine artisan.

The bone covering is made strong and firm by silica. In case of boils or carbuncle, the biochemist loses no time searching for "anthrax bacilli" or germs, nor does he experiment with imaginary germ-killing serum, but simply furnishes nature with tools with which the necessary work may be accomplished.

Silica gives the glossy finish to hair and nails. A stalk of corn or straw of wheat, oats or barley would not stand upright except they contained this mineral.

*This complete introductory section is adapted from:
The Chemistry and Wonders of the Human Body by Dr. George Carey.

MATERIA MEDICA FOR SILICEA

Adapted from: *The Biochemic System of Medicine, Materia Medica* by Dr. George Carey

The chemical action or function of silica as a worker in the human organism has never been clearly explained. Writers on biochemistry have hitherto fore been content to state its general action, and give it its place in the repertories according to certain symptoms. It is a constituent of common quartz, and found in the hair, nails, skin, periosteum, neurilemma, and a trace in the bone tissue. This salt is indicated in all suppurative processes until the infiltrated parts have fully discharged the heteroplasm or accumulation of decaying organic matter that may have arrived at a given point during nature's effort to eliminate it from the system. In the first stage of any swelling, Ferrum Phos and Kali Mur should be given (for reasons explained in biochemic pathology), but should these salts fail to abort the process, Silicea should at once be employed. When silica is present in proper quantities, the process of suppuration is carried on in a normal manner. When a deficiency of silica occurs, suppuration is retarded; the greater the deficiency, the greater and more stubborn and painful the swelling where the matter is attempting to escape, or, more correctly speaking, the point at which nature attempts to cast it off.

Characteristic Indications

(Note: The remedies in parentheses are support for Silicea.)

Mental symptoms – patient rather despondent and disgusted with life. Mental abstraction; difficulty of thought.

Head – Headache, when small lumps or nodules, about the size of a pea, appear on the scalp. **Scalp sensitive and sore to touch**. Painful pustules, suppurating wounds, with characteristic thick, yellow discharge of pus. Eruptions and nodules on the scalp; falling out of hair (Kali Sulph). **Sweat on head of children** also Calc Phos.

Eyes – Sty on the eyelid; internally and externally, to promote painless discharge of pus (if there is much inflammation, alternate Ferrum Phos). Disease of the lachrymal apparatus (tear duct). Lachrymal fistula (boil). Inflammations of the eye, with discharge of thick, yellow matter. Injuries of the eye, neglected cases, with subsequent suppuration of thick, yellow matter. Boils and indurations (hardenings) around eyelid. **Cataract after suppressed foot sweats or eruptions**.

Ears – Inflammatory swelling of external meatus (outer ear). Dullness of hearing, with swelling and **catarrh of the Eustachian tubes** and tympanic (inner ear) cavity. Boils and cystic tumors around the ear. Suppurative otitis (infected middle ear), when the discharge is thick, yellow matter. Otorrhea (inflamed ear canal), with caries (open wound) of the mastoid process (behind ear). Daily injections of the remedy – in water.

Nose – Catarrh of head, with characteristic discharge of fetid, thick, yellow matter. **Ozena** (bad smell from nose), when the affection is seated in the periosteum or in the sub-mucous connective tissues; **fetid, offensive discharge**. Nose, sore, with little boils around edges of nostrils, very itchy. Caries of the nasal bones, with very offensive discharge (Kali Phos). Dryness of the nostrils, with formation of scales and sores. Tip of nose red; itching of the tip of the nose.

Face – Face ache (trigeminal neuralgia), with small lumps or nodules on the face and scalp. Lupus, with discharge of thick matter. **Eruptions on the face**, from any cause, with discharge indicative of this remedy. Caries and necrosis of bones of the jaw. Induration of cellular tissues, after boils, etc.

Mouth – Suppurations of the glands of the mouth, with characteristic discharges.

Teeth – Toothache, very violent, at night, when neither heat nor cold gives relief, caused by chilling of the feet. **Toothache caused by sudden chilling of the feet when damp with perspiration.** Gumboils on the jaw. Toothache, with ulceration of the tooth; pain deep-seated in the periosteum.

Tongue – Hardening of the tongue. Ulcers on the tongue.

Throat – Ulcerations of the throat, with thick, yellow, mattery discharges. **Tonsillitis,** after pus has begun to form to produce suppuration; if it will not heal and infiltration has ceased, Calc Sulph is the remedy. Goiter.

Gastric symptoms – Induration of the pylorus (lower stomach valve). **Chronic dyspepsia** (poor digestion), with **acid eructations** (belching), with heartburn and chilliness (Nat Phos, Calc Phos). Child vomits as soon as it nurses; not sour (Ferrum Phos, Calc Phos).

Abdomen and stool – Abscess of the liver, with induration. **Sweating of the head in children,** with swollen abdomen and fetid, very offensive stools. Very painful piles (hemorrhoids), with discharges of thick, yellow matter. Fistula (boil-like) in anus, etc, with above symptoms.

Urinary organs – Suppurations (infections) of the kidneys, with urine loaded with pus and mucus. After febrile diseases, with the above discharges in the urine.

Male sexual organs – Chronic syphilis, with suppurations and hardening of the tissues. Prostatitis, when suppuration has commenced. Hydrocele (swollen testicles). Chronic gonorrhea, with thick, yellow, mattery discharges. **Itching of the scrotum with much sweat.**

Female sexual organs – Menses, when **associated with fetid sweating of the feet;** constipation; icy coldness all over the body. **Leucorrhea** (vaginal discharges), with characteristic discharge. **Metrorrhagia** (profuse menses) **from standing in cold water.** Abscess of the labia, with tendency to fistulous openings. Burning and itching of genital organs.

Pregnancy – Mastitis (inflamed breast), when

suppurating, to control the formation of pus (Kali Mur in first stage. Hard lumps in the breast, threatening suppuration (Kali Mur). **Fistulous ulcers of the breast,** with thick yellow discharge.

Respiratory organs – Inflammations of the respiratory tract, when tissue destruction has gone to that stage in which there is a copious expectoration of thick, yellow or greenish-yellow pus, accompanied with hectic fever, **profuse night sweats and great debility** (Calc Phos, Nat Mur). Consumption (tuberculosis), with the above symptoms. Abscess of the lungs, to promote suppuration and heal the ulcers, after suppuration has begun; sputa (saliva) abundant, thick and pus-like. Pneumonia, bronchitis, etc, suppurative stage (Calc Sulph).

Back and extremities – Neglected injuries, when festering or threatening to suppurate. Deep-seated wounds of the extremities, when discharging thick, yellow matter. **Hip-joint disease, to abort** or control **suppuration** and heal the parts. Whitlow (hangnails), to assist formation of pus and control suppuration, also to stimulate the growth of new nails (local application of the same). Carbuncles, boil-like (after Kali Mur), to mature the tumor and discharge matter. **Foul perspiration of the feet,** very offensive smell. Caries of the bone, with fistulous openings; discharging pus; if bony fragments, alternate Calc Fluor. Psoas (groin muscle) abscess, Pott's disease (spinal bone destruction).

Nervous symptoms – Obstinate neuralgia, occurring at night, when neither heat nor cold gives relief. Epilepsy and **spasms occurring at night,** or from slight provocation; very obstinate cases (Mag Phos, Calc Phos, Kali Mur). (Cuprum Met)

Skin – Inflammation of, or injuries to, the skin, at that stage when thick, yellow pus is being discharged. **Tendency to boils** in any part of the body, especially **in the springtime.** Carbuncles, boils, ulcers, felons, etc., if deep-seated and discharging thick, heavy, yellow pus. Skin heals slowly and suppurates easily after injuries. Ulcers around nails, with unhealthy-looking skin. Scrofulous (dirty looking) eruption. Pustules on face and neck; extremely painful. Leprosy, for the nasal ulceration, nodes (round swelling) and coppery spots.

Tissues – Abscess, easily bleeding after matter has begun to form, chief remedy, to promote the discharge of pus (Kali Mur, before matter forms). Swellings of the glands (if Kali Mur does not abort them and matter has formed). **Suppurating glands, with thick yellow, offensive discharge** of matter. Scrofulous, enlarged glands. Neglected cases of injury, with suppuration. Ulceration and caries of bone. Malignant, gangrenous inflammation (Kali Phos).

Silicea Summary

ORGAN AND TISSUE AFFINITIES
Connective tissue, bones, skin, nutrition, nerves, glands, cartilage.

MODALITIES
Symptoms worse < cold air, drafts, head uncovered, nervous excitement, new moon, milk, menses, night.
Symptoms better > warmth, urination, wrapping the head tightly.

DEFICIENCY SYMPTOMS
Sweaty hands and feet, stinky feet, light and noise sensitivity, dry brittle nails, splinters, skin problems in general, shy person, cold body, smelly armpits..

DISEASE CONDITIONS
Splinters, keloids (raised scars), vaccination reactions, emaciation, exhaustion, pus formation, skin problems.

Febrile conditions – **Copious night sweats, with prostration** in phthisis (tuberculosis), or when no other disease is apparent. **Sweat about the head in children.** Hectic fever, with burning in soles of feet. **Offensive sweat of feet and armpits.** Fever during suppurative processes.

Sleep – Sleeplessness from excess of blood; **wakefulness in old people**, with phthisis. **Jerking of limbs during sleep.**

Modalities – Symptoms are always worse at night. Better by heat and in warm room. **Worse from chilling of the feet.** Worse in open air.

FACIAL SIGNS OF SILICEA DEFICIENCY

Wrinkles are a big sign of Silicea deficiency. Silicea is very important in connective tissue development. A silicea deficiency is often seen in shrunken connective tissue that shows up in facial wrinkles etc. The wrinkles are signs of early old age. The wrinkles are more often seen in the corners of the eyes, forehead, cheeks, and in front on the ears.

Wrinkles in front of and parallel to the ears are another sign. These wrinkles are vertical above the upper lip and seen by many as liquid problems but doesn't relate to this problem. The wrinkles come about from connective tissue weakness where the tissue shrinks and enlarges. The folds first gather and enlarge parallel to the ears. This can be seen in young people and with enough silicea can be reversed. The first sign of silicea is seen in the wrinkles parallel to the ears and can extend further on the face as the deficiency deepens.

Laugh lines and crow's feet show a deeper deficiency, we see the laugh lines on the corners of the eyes and further deficiency deepens them as they become crows feet and can extend to the cheeks and the chin.

Eyelid cavity/eye orbits of the connective tissue of the upper eyelids are shrunken and the lid

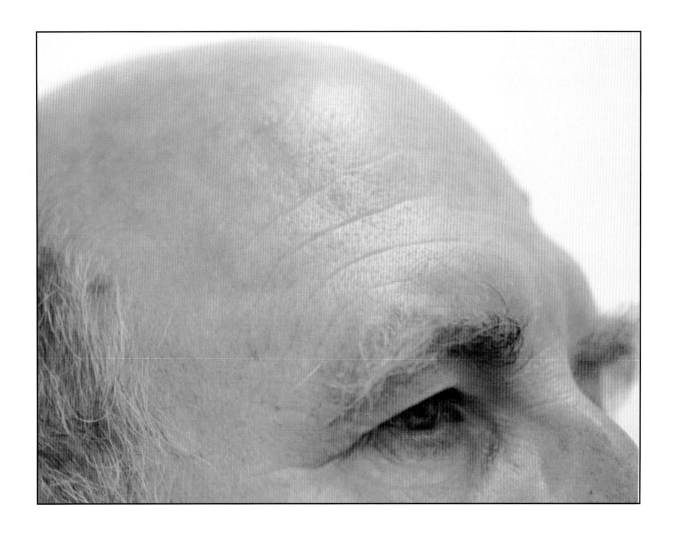

Silicea (a)

This man's head has the polished shine of a Silicea deficiency. He also has the Silicea deep-set eyes and a shiny nose. There is a slight waxy appearance around the eyebrows that shows a Calc Phos deficiency.

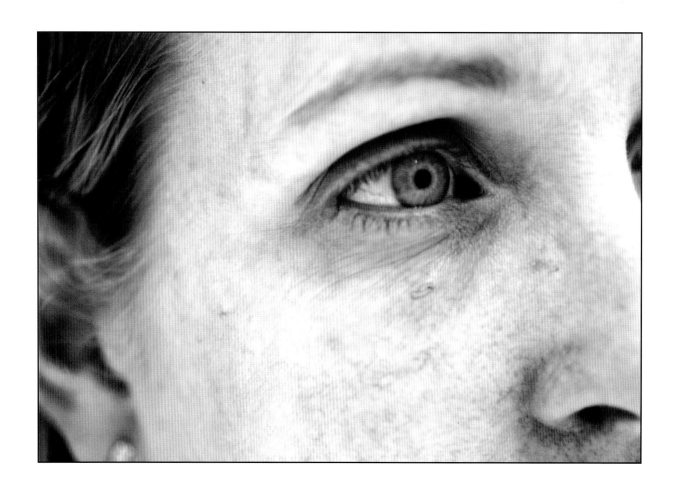

Silicea (b)

The Silicea deficiency seen here is in the translucent skin quality of the temple area. There are also the beginnings of fan-shaped wrinkles that start from the corner of the eye, with dark circles under the eye, indicating a Calc Fluor deficiency. There is a green shading indicative of a Nat Sulph deficiency. The reddish coloring next to the nose is a Kali Mur deficiency.

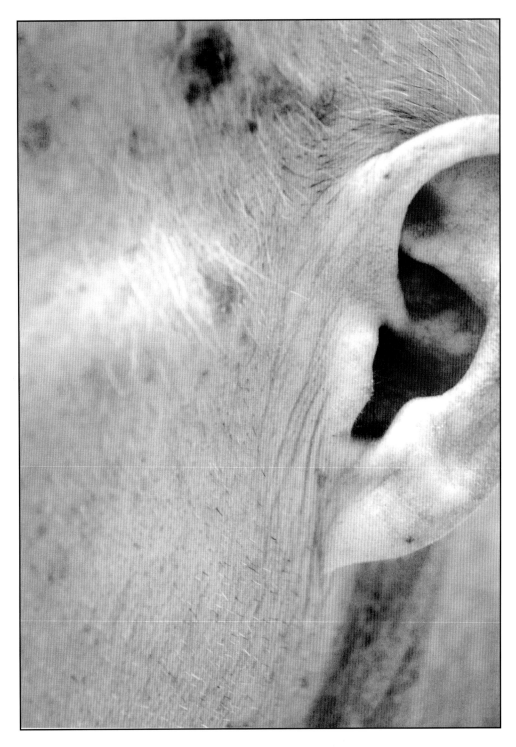

Silicea (c)

The parallel lines next to the ear are signs of a Silicea deficiency. The greenish tinge indicates a liver problem and is a Nat Sulph deficiency sign. The milky red of the earlobe is a Kali Mur deficiency symptom.

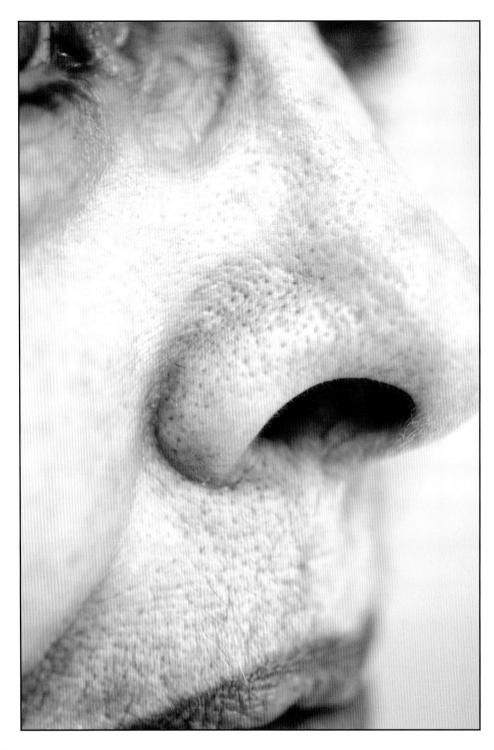

Silicea (d)

This woman's nose has the polished shine of a Silicea deficiency. This nose has large pores – showing a Nat Mur deficiency. The area below the nose has the vertical lines of a Nat Phos deficiency, which indicates an acid condition in the body.

looks very deeply indented. There is an empty space in the orbit area.

Glassy or polished shine is a reflective shine of Calc Fluor, and a greasy shine of Nat Mur. The Silicea shine is characterized by the shine of the typical bald head. It is a shine of the outer skin, and a translucent skin appearance. Frequently this shine is seen on the forehead by the hairline.

Split hair ends are often a sign of Silicea deficiency. This is often an acidity problem and a mineral deficiency. The hair no longer has a shine and splits easily. This is often seen with a Nat Phos deficiency and can be seen on the tongue.

The person with Silicea deficiency often is light sensitive and must wear sunglasses. (Nat Mur)

Burst veins in whites of eyes. When the arterial walls of the blood vessels are weak, they can burst and have a reddened appearance. One can see easy bruising in the elderly or there can be other problems such as high blood pressure, overwork, or alcohol use. (Arnica)

Nail problems are seen. Even though this is not a facial sign, silicea deficiency is seen in soft, weak, splitting nails.

THERAPEUTIC INDEX FOR SILICEA

Adapted from: *Therapeutic Index* (1890) by Dr. W. H. Schuessler

Boils, little lumps, not mattery. (Hepar Sulph)

Chilblains (frostbite), festering, as second remedy.

Ear, swelling, inflammatory, of the external meatus.

Epilepsy, nocturnal fits, at the changes of the moon.

Face ache (trigeminal neuralgia) with concurrent appearance of small nodules, lumps the size of a pea on scalp.

Glands, suppurating, if Calc Sulph is not suitable.

Headaches, with concurrent appearance of small lumps, nodules size of a pea on scalp.

Hip joint disease, controls suppuration during that process.

Injuries, neglected cases, if suppurating.

Intermittent fever, some species of .

Mastitis, during suppuration, to control the formation of pus.

Secretions, mattery, bloody mattery.

Skin affections, dry eruptions with corresponding symptoms.

Suppurations, pus, infection, festers, having their seat in the cell-substance of the connective tissue. All such suppurations, including those of bone, are cured by this remedy.

Suppurations of joints, to control the formation of pus.

Tongue, indurations of.

ASTROLOGY OF SILICEA
The Chemistry of Sagittarius
November 22 to December 22

Adapted from: *Cell Salts of Salvation* by Dr. George Carey

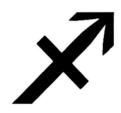 The mineral or cell salt of the blood corresponding to Sagittarius is silica (Silicia). This salt is the surgeon of the human organism. The centaur of mythology is known in the "Circles of Beasts that worship before the Lord (Sun) day and night," as Sagittarius, the Archer, with drawn bow. Arrowheads are composed of flint, de-carbonized white pebble or quartz. Thus we see why Silicea is a special birth-salt of all born in the Sagittarius sign.

Sagittarius people are generally swift and strong; and they are prophetic – look deeply into the future and hit the mark like the archer. A

noted astrologer once said: "Never lay a wager with one born with the Sun in Sagittarius or with Sagittarius rising in the east lest you lose your wealth."

The Sagittarius native is very successful in thought transference. He (or she) can concentrate on a brain, miles distant, and so vibrate the aerial wires that fill space that the molecular intelligence of these finely attuned to nature's harmonies may read the message.

The governing planet of Sagittarius is Jupiter. Its associated gems are carbuncle, diamond and turquoise, and its astral colors are gold, red and green. Sagittarius is a fire sign and is represented in Bible alchemy by Levi, the third son of Jacob, meaning "joined or associated." In the symbolism of New Testament, Sagittarius corresponds with the disciple James, son of Alpheus.

Appendix

The worksheet that follows on page 152 is designed to give the practitioner an easy reference for the uses of the cell salts by noting the prominent facial signs. It is a place to record observations and the recommended doses given to any patient.

Facial Analysis for:

Address: Birthdate:

Cell Salt	Facial Signs	# salts	# salts	# salts	# salts	# salts
1. Calc Fluor	Blue lips, brownish-black color, white flakes, translucent tips of teeth, reflective shine –especially in acute situations. Raised and/or fan-shaped wrinkles, furrows, cracked lips.					
2. Calc Phos	White waxy appearance, translucent tips of teeth, white flakes in teeth or fingernails, stretched skin on cheekbones, small lips.					
3. Calc Sulph	Alabaster or pale white coloring, mainly on the lower face and jaw					
4. Ferr Phos	Bluish-black shade, red ears, shading in corner of the eyes, furrows, hung-over or sleepless appearance, inflamed skin.					
5. Kali Mur	Milky red, blue or purple skin, acne rosacea, red spider veins, chicken skin.					
6. Kali Phos	Ashen gray appearance, frosted look of eyes, sunken temples and/or cheeks, bad breath.					
7. Kali Sulph	Brownish-yellow ocher pigmentation, liver spots, age spots, vitilago, freckles, pregnancy mask.					
8. Mag Phos	Redness (chronic), nerve spots, alcohol redness.					
9. Nat Mur	Gelatinous, often on the upper eyelid or the edge of the eyelashes on the lower lid, red border at the hairline, inflamed eyelids, large pores, dandruff, dry skin, puffy cheeks, spongy or bloated appearance, bell-shaped nose, sweat, greasy skin.					
10. Nat Phos	Greasy, it has a greasy feel too, combination skin, cholesterol deposits (raised yellow, pimple-like growths around the eyes), red chin, acid spots, dry skin, dry or greasy hair, greasy sweat.					
11. Nat Sulph	Greenish-yellow coloring, bluish-red, yellowish sclera, swollen lower eyelid sacks, bad smelling gas.					
12. Silicea	Glassy or polished-shine look, wrinkles in general, vertical wrinkles parallel to the ears, laugh lines, crows feet, deep eyelids, split ends on hair, fingernail problems, red eyes (burst veins of the eyeballs).					

Glossary

Albumen – egg-white–like protein. *Also* albuminous, albuminoid.

Anteversion – tipped uterus.

Arteritis – inflammation of the artery.

Articular – joint-related.

Asthenic – weak, exhausted.

Atrophic – wasting of tissues, organs or entire body.

Bilious – (relating to bile), congestive disturbance with coated tongue, headache, dizziness, assumed to result from hepatic function.

Blebs – small blister or pustule.

Blind headache – causes partial or total temporary loss of sight.

Bright's disease – kidney disease of albuminous kind.

Bubo – swelling of the lymph glands, especially in the groin.

Carbuncle – boil.

Caries – ulceration of bone, resembling gangrene of soft parts, most commonly caused by blows to bone, or some virus.

Catarrh – mucus congestion. *Also* catarrhal.

Cerebritis – inflammation of the cerebrum.

Chancre – syphilitic or hard ulcer, begins as a papule and breaks down into an ulcer.

Chilblains – frostbite of the hands and feet with burning and itching, sometimes chapping and ulceration.

Chlorosis – condition giving greenish tinge to the skin. *Also* chlorotic.

Cholera – bilious disease term, non-specific for a variety of gastrointestinal disturbances causing a profuse watery diarrhea, extreme loss of fluid and electrolytes, and a state of collapse.

Chorea – involuntary limb movement or St. Vitus' dance

Consumption – wasting of the tissues of the body, usually referred to as tuberculosis.

Coryza – cold in head.

Costiveness – constipation.

Crusta lactea (cradle cap) – condition afflicting infants and little children that creates Scaly crusts on the scalp.

Cystitis – inflammation of the bladder.

Delirium tremens – shaking caused by alcohol withdrawal.

Desquamation – destruction of the skin.

Diphtheria – an infectious disease marked by inflammation with formation of a fibrinous exudate of the mucus membranes of the throat and nose.

Diplopia – double vision.

Dropsy – swelling.

Dysentery – a disease marked by frequent watery stools, often with blood and mucus, characterized by pain, tenesmus, fever and dehydration.

Dysmenorrhea – painful menstruation.

Dyspepsia – indigestion.

Embolus – blood clot

Encephalitis – inflammation of the brain.

Enteric fever – typhoid and paratyphoid fevers.

Enuresis – urinary incontinence.

Epigastrium – upper- middle region of the abdomen.

Epistaxis – nosebleed.

Epithelium – skin or membrane. *Also* epithelial.

Eruptive fever – *see* typhus.

Erysipelas – redness of the skin from inflammation. *Also* erysipelatous.

Exuberant granulation – a fungus growth from a granulating surface that shows no tendency of scar formation.

Exudation – the process of exuding or oozing.

False Diphtheria – (pseudo diphtheria), one of a group of local infections, suggesting diphtheria caused by microorganisms other than *diphtheria bacillus.*

Febrile – pertaining to fever.

Felon – infected hangnail.

Festers – small festering sores or ulcers.

Fibrin – fibrous protein. *Also* fibrinous.

Fistulous – pertaining to an abnormal passage leading from an abscessed cavity or hollow organ to the surface, or to another cavity or organ.

Flatus – gas.

Florid – complexion of bright red color: denoting certain skin changes or injury.

Fungoid – resembling fungus.

Furuncles – boils.

Gastric derangement – digestive problem in which trapped gas applies pressure on the lungs.

Glairy – viscous substance resembling egg-white.

Gleet – chronic inflammation of a bodily orifice.

Glottis – vocal apparatus of the larynx, including vocal cords.

Goiter – chronic enlargement of the thyroid gland.

Gonorrhea – a contagious catarrhal inflammation of the genital mucus membrane, transmitted by coitus.

Griping – colic, sharp pain in the bowels.

Hectic fever – characterized by irritation and debility, occurring usually at the advanced stage of an exhausting disease, as in pulmonary consumption.

Heteroplasm – dissimilar tissue.

Hemiplegia – paralysis of one side of the body.

Housemaid's knee – swelling of the knee.

Hydrocephalus – water in the head.

Hydroma patella – swelling of the kneecap.

Hydrops – swelling.

Hyperemia – accumulation of blood in any of the blood vessels.

Ichorous – pertaining to a watery, acrid discharge from wound or ulcer.

Idiopathic – denoting a disease of unknown
.

Induration – hardening.

Infiltrations – growths infiltrating into the tissue of the joints or hair follicles.

Inguinal – related to the groin area.

Inspissation – act or the process of inspissating, or thickening a fluid substance, as by evaporation; also, the state of being so thickened.

Intercurrent remedy – using another cell salt when the healing process has stalled; once there is movement, go back to the original remedy.

Intermittent fever – fever with marked intervals, resembling malaria, with absence of symptoms between paroxysms.

Intertrigo – an inflammation of the top layers of skin caused by moisture, bacteria, or fungi in the folds of the skin.

Ischuria – suppression of urine.

Jaundice – yellowness caused by hepatic dysfunction.

Lachrymation – shedding of tears.

Lachrymose – depressive.

Leucorrhea – discharge from the vagina.

Lockjaw – firm closing of the jaw due to tonic spasms of muscles, associated and due to general tetanus.

Marasmus – failure to thrive.

Mastitis – inflammation of the breast.

Mattery – pus-containing.

Meningitis – inflammation of the membranes of the brain or spinal cord.

Metritis – inflammation of the uterus.

Naevi – moles.

Necrosis – the pathological death of one or more cells or a portion of tissues or organ, resulting from irreversible damage.

Nettle rash – stinging rash.

Orchitis – testicle inflammation.

Ostitis – bone inflammation.

Ozeana – condition with foul-smelling nasal discharge.

Paralysis agitans – Parkinson's disease, shaking palsy.

Paresis – slight or partial paralysis

Paroxysms – sharp spasm or convulsion. Sudden onset of a symptom of disease especially with recurrent manifestations such as chills and rigor of malaria.

Pedunculated – as if on a stalk.

Pemphigus – eruption of blister.

Pericarditis – inflammation of pericardium.

Periosteum – bone covering.

Periostitis – inflammation of bone covering.

Peritonitis – inflammation of membrane that lines the abdominal cavity.

Phagedenic – rapidly spreading, destroying tissues as it increases in size.

Phthisis – a wasting or atrophy, local or general.

Pleura – mucus membrane enveloping the lung.

Pleurisy – inflammation of the membrane that envelops the lungs.

Polyuria simplex – excessive secretion of urine.

Prolapsus – falling down or slipping out of place of an organ or part.

Proud flesh – a fungus growth from a granulating surface that shows no tendency of scar formation.

Pruritis – itching.

Puerperal – postpartum.

Purulent – pus-filled.

Quinsy – inflammation of the tonsils.

Remittent fever – a malarial fever in which temperature falls more or less, but not to normal, between two paroxysms.

Retroversion – bending backwards of the uterus.

Rheumatic fever – fever occurring during recovery from infection, usually of the throat.

Rheumatism – various conditions with pain or other symptoms, which are of articular (joint) origin or related to other elements of the musculoskeletal system.

Rickets – calcium deficiency disease characterized by softening of bones with associated skeletal deformities.

Rupia – cysts under tongue.

Sanious – watery and blood-tinged, foul.

Sciatica – neuralgia of the sciatic nerve, either due to herniated lumbar disc, or sciatic neuritis.

Scrofula – swelling of the lymph nodes. *Also* scrofulous.

Serous – resembling serum.

Spermatorrhea – involuntary discharge of semen, without orgasm.

Sputa – spit.

St. Vitus's dance – chorea.

Stitching – sticking pain of momentary duration.

Stomatitis – cankers.

Subcutaneous – below the skin; hypodermic.

Suppuration – discharge of pus from infection.

Sycosis – inflammation of the hair follicles.

Syncope – fainting.

Syphilis – acute or chronic infectious disease transmitted by direct contact, usually through sexual intercourse.

Tabes dorsalis – wasting of the spinal cord.

Tabes mesenterica – abdominal lymph-wasting disease.

Tic-douloureux – facial tics.

Tinnitis aurium – sensation of noise in the ears.

Tracheitis – inflammation of the trachea.

Tubercles – nodules.

Tuberculosis – a disease that may affect almost any tissue or organ of the body, the most common seat of the disease is in the lungs. General symptoms are those of sepsis: hectic fever, sweats, and emaciation.

Tympanitis – inflammation of the inner ear.

Typhus – an acute infectious or contagious disease. Usually marked by high fever, mental and physical depression, and macular and papular eruption, lasting up to two weeks. Also called camp fever.

Uvula – fleshy mass of tissue suspended from the center of the soft palate.

Varicocele – a varicose condition of veins of the spermatic cord, forming a soft tumor.

Vesicles – blisters

Vitiligo – lack of pigmentation in skin.

Wasting disease – emaciation.

Whitlow – infected hangnails.

Yellow fever – a mosquito-borne viral hepatitis characterized by fever, slow pulse, albuminaria, congestion of the face, and hemorrhages.

Bibliography

GERMAN

Emmrich, Peter, *Antlitzdiagnostik*. Neckersulm, Germany: Jungjohann Verlag, 2003.

Keller, Georg, Ulrike Novotny, and Markus Wiesenauer, *12 Salze 12 Typen*. Munich, Germany: Weltbild Ratgeber Verlag, 2002.

Tichy, E. and K. Tichy, *Das grosse Praxisbuch der Schuesslertherapie*. Stuttgart, Germany: Johannes Sonntag Verlagsbuchhandlung, 2001.

Feichtinger, Thomas, Elisabeth Mandl, and Susana Niedan, *Handbuch der Biochemie nach Dr. Schuessler*. Heidelberg, Germany: Karl R. Haug Verlage, 2002.

Feichtinger, Thomas and Susana Niedan, *Antlitzdiagnostik in der Biochemie nach Dr. Schuessler*. Stuttgart, Germany: Karl F. Haug Verlage, 2002.

Schleimer, J., *Salze des Lebens*. Regensburg, Germany: Johannes Sonntag, 1984.

ENGLISH

Carey, George W., *The Chemistry and Wonders of the Human Body*. Los Angeles: The Chemistry of Life Co., 1963.

Carey, George W., *The Biochemic System of Medicine*. Calcutta, India: A.P. Homeolibrary, Sri H.Dey, 1962.

Carey, George W., *The Zodiac and the Salts of Salvation*. York Beach, Maine: Samuel Weiser, Inc., 1996.

Boerice, William and W.A. Dewey, *The Twelve Tissue Remedies of Schuessler*. New Delhi, India: B. Jain Publishers, 1992.

Chapman, J.B. and J.W. Cogswell, *Dr. Schuessler's Biochemistry, a New Domestic Treatise*. St. Louis: Luyties Pharmacal Company.

Schuessler, W. H., *New Treatment of Disease*. Edinburgh and Glasgow, Scotland: John Mensies & Co., 1880.

Cell Salt Sources

Dave's Health & Nutrition
3 locations. We can ship anywhere.
You may also fax your orders to any store.

1108 E. 3300 S., Salt Lake City, Utah, (801) 483-9024, Fax (801) 483-9052

7777 S. State Street, Midvale, Utah, (801) 255-3809, Fax (801) 566-2725

1817 W. 9000 S, West Jordan, Utah, (801) 446-0499, Fax (801) 446-0582

Boiron
Simi Valley, California, (800) 373-6633

Dolisos
Las Vegas, Nevada, (800) 365-4767

Standard Homeopathics
Los Angeles, California, (800) 624-9659

Cell salts are available in bottles of 250 – 4,000 count.
Cell salts of 6x potency are available in 500 and 1,000 count bottles.

Index

A

abdominal sagging, 18
abscesses, 41, 144. *See also* suppuration
acid balance, 120
acid conditions, 14, 120, 121. *See also*
   indigestion
acne, 29, 66. *See also* pimples
   blackheads, 6, 14, 123
   rosacea, 4, 6, 31, 67
age spots, 4, 42, 90
air, open, 66, 89, 128, 144
alcohol 6, 135
allergies, 66
anal fissure, 19, 30
anemia, 32, 78
aneurysm, 19, 53
angina pectoris, 100
ankles, weak, 32
antispasmodic remedy, 97
anxiety, 29, 76
appetite 30, 64, 77
arthritis. *See* rheumatism
ash-gray appearance, 6
asthma, 80
   bronchial, 77, 88
   chest soreness and, 53
   cough and, 19, 99, 110, 133
   damp wet conditions and, 133
   gas/belching, with, 99
   gastric derangement, from, 65
   labored breathing and, 77
   violent attacks of, 133
astrology, *See* zodiac
atrophy, of organ tissue, 32

B

back
   coldness in, 11
   pain (backache) in, 19, 53, 100, 111
   rheumatism in, 31, 53, 133
bags under eyes, 4

bald(ness), 4, 29
ball, rising in the throat, 77
bathing, 41
bed wetting, 37, 52, 77
belching, 30, 52, 64, 99
bile, 64, 121, 130, 132, 133
bilious disorders, 121, 133. *See also*
   indigestion
biochemistry, definition of, 10
blackheads. *See under* acne
bladder
   inflammation in, 41, 52
   spasm of, 99
   stones, prevention of, 30
bleeding, 54, 85
blisters, 66, 78, 111, 117
bloated appearance, 6, 112
bloating, of abdomen, 88, 99
blood
   acid conditions of, 120
   clots in brain, 25
   clotting of, 39
   hemoglobin, 54
   hemorrhage, 51
   loss of, causing swelling, 54
blood vessels, 18, 53
blue shading, 4
bluish black, 4, 55
bluish-red color, 4
blushing, acute, 4
body temperature 25, 112, 144
boils, 14, , 42, 143
bone growth, 14
bones
   broken, 31, 37, 55
   bruises to, 20
   building of, 27
   constituents of, 10
   diseases of, 27, 31, 32
   infections of, 20
   inflammation of, 60

bones (cont.)
  nutrition of, 32
  pains in, 31
  rugged surface of, 25
  ulcerations of, 18
  weak, 31
bowels, 19, 41, 67
bowlegs, 31
brain,
  blood clots in the, 25
  cells, 74
  concussion, 80
  congestion of, 51
  fatigue from overwork, 75
  fevers, 79
  swelling, 29
  water on the, 37
breast(s)
  inflammation of, 53
  knots in, 19, 25
  lumps, 143
  pus discharging from, 41
  ulcers, 143
breath, bad (offensive), 6, 14, 76, 80
Bright's disease, 30, 55, 77
bronchitis, 110, 117, 133, 143
brown to yellow, color around mouth, 4
brownish yellow appearance, 4, 6, 89
brownish-black, 4, 20
bruises, 66
bubo, 65
burns, 42, 63, 66
businessman, 75

C
caffeine, 3
Calc Phos (calcium fluoride), 17
  Astrology of, Cancer, 25
  Deficiency Symptoms, 25
  Disease Conditions, 25
  Facial Signs of Deficiency, 20
  hardening of the tissues and, 17
  Materia Medica, 18
  Modalities, 25
  Organ and Tissue Affinities, 25
  relaxed conditions of elastic fiber
    and, 17
  Summary, 25
  Therapeutic Index, 25
Calc Phos (calcium phosphate), 27
  Astrology of, Capricorn, 38
  as bone builder, 27
  Bright's disease and, 27
  Deficiency Symptoms, 32
  Disease Conditions, 32
  Facial Signs of Deficiency, 32
  Materia Medica, 28
  Modalities, 32

  Organ and Tissue Affinities, 32
  restorative, as a, 31
  Summary, 32
  Therapeutic Index, 32
Calc Sulph (calcium sulphate), 39
  Astrology of, Scorpio, 47
  Deficiency Symptoms, 41
  Disease Conditions, 41
  Facial Signs of Deficiency, 42
  Materia Medica, 40
  Modalities, 41
  mucus congestion, and, 39
  Organ and Tissue Affinities, 41
  skin tissue and 39
  Summary, 41
  suppuration and, 39
  Therapeutic Index, 42
calcium fluoride, See Calc Fluor
calcium phosphate, See Calc Phos
calcium sulphate, See Calc Sulph
calves, cramps in, 100
cancer, 37
  epithelial (skin) 89
  face, 88
  lips, 88
  nose, 88
candida, 128
cankers, 51, 64, 76
cartilage, 32
cataracts, 18, 87, 142
cell salts
  astrology and, 6-8
  bases available in, 1
  facial locations of deficiencies of, 4-6
  history of, 10
  products that reverse action of, 3
  storage of, 2
  use and handling of, 1-3
cephalhematoma, 25
changing symptoms, 14
chattering teeth. See under teeth
cheeks
  hamster appearance, 128
  hot, 51
  puffy, 6, 112
  red, 4
  sunken, 4, 6
  swelling of, 19, 64
cheekbones, stretched skin on, 6, 32
chest, 31, 88
chest pain, from coughing, 111
chicken skin, 6, 67
chicken pox, 54
chilblains, 65, 78, 149
children
  asthma in, 134
  bed wetting of, 77
  colic in, 99, see also gas

convulsions in, 31, 53, 99
cradle cap (crusta lactea) of, 66
crossness of, 75
epileptic fits in, 37
failure to thrive, of, 30
fever. See under fever
growing pains in, 14
head tumors in infants, 18
headaches in, 14, 55
ill-tempered, 76
neck thin in, 31
nosebleeds of, 55
nursing of, 30, 31
pale face of, 29
screaming during sleep, 76
skin, chafing of, 111
sleepwalking by, 76
stools of. See stools
sweat on head of, 142
teeth-grinding of, during sleep, 122
teething of, 4, 29, 30, 52, 53, 109, 122
thrush in, 67, 109
vomiting of, 31
chills, 100, 112, 130, 140
chilliness, 32, 87, 112
chin, 4, 6, 128
chlorosis, 32
chocolate cravings, 14
choking, 99
cholera, 80
circles under eyes, 4
circulation, poor, 31, 111
coccyx, injuries of, 31
coffee, effects on cell salts, 3
cold damp, 25, 32, 54
cold drinks, 30, 66
cold sores, 14, 65
colds, 29, 50, 53, 88, 109
  chest. See respiratory tract
  head, 14, 18, 28, 29, 64, 67, 88
  nasal discharge, see nose
colic, 101. See also gas; indigestion
collapse, 80
colon, peristalsis, 100
color of skin. See skin
concussion. See under brain
congestion, 37. See also colds
conjunctivitis, 87, 109, 132
connective tissue, 13
constellations, 2
constipation, 30, 52, 64, 110
cornea problems, 14, 25, 40, 42, 67,
  109
cough, 55, 67. See also hawking
  chest pain from, 111
  convulsive fits of, 100
  cool air and, 88
  dry, 53

evening and, 88
expectoration,
   clear and thick, 31
     lumpy, 19
     white, 65
     yellow sputa, 88
   hoarseness, with, 65
   spasmodic, 65, 78, 100
   tear flow, with, 111
   tickling, 19
   whooping, chief remedy for, 85
   "winter cough," 110
cradle cap. *See under* children
cramping, remedy for, 100
cramps, muscular, 97
croup, 42, 55, 65
crow's feet. *See under* wrinkles
cuts, swollen, 66
cystitis, 55, 65. *See also* bladder

D

dampness, 66
dandruff, 6, 87, 112, 90, 109
deafness 51, 63, 87, 109
debility, 78, 143
decaying matter, discharge of, 141
delirium tremens, 107
delirium, 55, 109
depression, 29, 75, 79, 134
dermatitis, contact, 41
despondent moods, 109, 132, 142
diabetes insipidus, 110
diabetes mellitus, 37, 77, 128, 133
diarrhea, 77
   bilious, 12, 135
   dark greenish, 133
   mattery, bloody, 42
   straining at stool and, 122
   yellow, 64, 88
digestion, 28, 30, 117, 121, 128. *See also* indigestion
diphtheria, 37, 64, 80, 117, 122
dirty-looking face, 29, 42
Discharges Indicative of Cell Salt Deficiencies, 16
discharges. *See also* specific body part
   blood-stained, 41
   clear, 14
   menstrual. *See under* menstrual
   nasal. *See under* nose
   pus, 20, 39
   vaginal. *See* leucorrhea
   watery, 14, 107, 109
   white, 14, 63, 65
   yellow 14, 18, 42, 87, 123, 142
disease, 10-12
disgust with life, 142
dizziness, 76

dosage of cell salts 1
doubling over, condition better by, 41
dread, 76
dreams, 32, 134
drinks. *See* cold drinks, hot drinks
dysentery, 77, 99
dysmenorrhea. *See under* menses
dyspepsia, 52, 88, 110, 122, 128, 143. *See also* gas

E

ear(s)
   canal, inflamed, 142
   cracking noises on blowing nose, 63
   discharges,
     clear thick, 29
     foul, offensive, 76
     gray, thick, 63
     mixed with blood, 76
     yellow, 87, 122
   diseases of, 18
   eustachian tubes and, 14, 87, 142
   hearing and, dullness of, 76, 98, 142
   inner, 51, 63
   itching of, 29
   lobes, paleness of, 55
   middle, 142
   outer, 4, 29, 32, 51, 122
earache, 29, 51, 55, 63, 87, 98, 132
eating, red nose after, 128
eczema, 31, 37, 41, 66, 78, 111, 123
   See also skin
edema. *See* swelling
electrical shock, 31
elements, the four, 6
emaciate(d), 30, 111, 112, 144
Emotional Symptoms of Cell Salt Deficiencies, 15
enamel, of teeth. *See under* teeth
encephalitis, 72
enuresis, nocturnal, 37, 52, 77
epilepsy, 53, 66, 78, 100, 143
eruptions. See specific body part
eustachian tubes. *See under* ears
exhaustion, 79, 100
extremities, ulcers in, 65
eyeballs ache, 29
eyebrows, 4, 32
eye(s)
   conjunctiva of, 6, 132
   corners, shading of, 6
   deep-set, 6, 148-149
   discharges of,
     clear, 109
     white, 63
     yellow 40, 122, 142
     yellow-greenish, 87
   dull-looking, 4

   frosted look of, 6, 80
   glued together in morning, 122
   inflammation of, 29, 40, 51, 63
   lids, *see* eyelids
   pain in, 51, 98, 109
   resting of, 18
   sacks under, 6, 135
   sight, loss of, 29
   sore, 63
   sunken, 144
   tear duct(s) of, 142
   tears, 109
   whites of, 149
   yellow sclera of, 6
eyelids, 6, 29
   burning of, 132
   crusts, yellow, 87
   drooping, 76, 98
   flaking off, upper, 20
   granulated, 51, 63
   spasmodic, 37, 98
eyesight, 85

F

face. *See also* skin
   cancer, 88
   dirty-looking, 29
   eruptions, 29, 142
   flushed, 51
   herpes on, 111, 117
   hung-over appearance of, 6, 55
   liver spots on, 4, 42
   neuralgia of, 76, 88
   pains in, 29, 99. *See also* faceache
   perspiration on, while eating, 109
   red and blotched, without fever, 122
   redness of, 132
   rheumatism of, 29
   sunken, 76
   sweat, 32
   swollen, due to alcohol, 112
   whiskers, 109
   yellow, 132
face ache, 37, 55, 64, 142
fainting 76, 78
fat digestion, problems with, 66
fears, of financial ruin, 17
feet, 14, 35
   perspiration of, 25, 143
   soles of, 41
   swelling of, 65
   twitching during sleep, 134
Ferrum Phos (iron phosphate), 49
   Astrology of, Pisces, 60
   Deficiency Symptoms, 54
   Disease Conditions, 54
   Facial Signs of Deficiency, 54
   fevers, all, 49

Ferrum Phos (cont.)
inflammatory Symptoms, 49
iron, deficiency of, 49
Materia Medica, 50
Modalities, 54
Organ and Tissue Affinities, 54
oxygen, affinity for, 49
Summary, 54
Therapeutic Index, 55
fever, 49, 55, 79, 140
intermittent, 37, 42, 134
postpartum, 65, 77
stages of, 14
types of, 132
fibroids, 14
fingernail problems. *See* nails
fingers, 47, 53, 100, 117
fits, from fright, 80
flakes, white, 4. *See also* skin
flatulence, 77, 122. *See also* gas
fluids, loss of, 32
fontanelles, 29, 37
food, non-assimilation of, 30
Foods Rich in Cell Salt Nutrients, 14
fractures, first remedy for, 55. *See also*
bones
freckles, 4, 31, 90
frostbite. *See* chilblains
furrows. *See under* wrinkles

G
gallstones, prevention of, 30
gangrenous conditions, 79
gas, 121, 122, 133. *See also* flatulence
acid condition and, 29
belching. *See under* belching
caused by hot drinks, 64
during menstrual periods, 77
smell of, 6, 14, 88, 135
glands
around ears, 63
enlarged, 37
hardened, 18
inflammation of, 111, 117, 144
suppuration of, 42
under tongue, 109
Glauber's salts, 131
gloomy moods, 76
goiter, 29, 143
gonorrhea, 30, 65, 110
gout, 111, 123, 133
gray coloring, in face, 4
greasy food, 64
green coloring, 4
greenish tint, 37
greenish-white complexion, 32
greenish-yellow color, 4, 6, 135
grief, desire for solitude after, 29

grievances, dwells upon, 78
groin abscess, 143
growth, stunted, 32
growths, on bone surfaces, 20
gumboil, 64, 143
gums, 51, 76, 79

H
hairline, redness of, 4, 112
hair follicles, inflammation of, 66
hair
brittle, 14
glossy finish to, 141
greasy, 6, 14
loss of, 29, 87
split ends, 6, 14, 149
hands,
blisters on, 111
chapped, 20, 67
cold, poor circulation in, 111
involuntary motion of, 100
perspiration on, 31
swollen, 14
twitching during sleep, 134
warts, on palms of, 111
hangnails, 20, 47, 53, 78, 111, 143
hardening of the tissues, 17
hawking, 29, 31, 133. *See also* cough
hay fever, 77, 109
head cold. *See under* colds
head, 18, 29, 76, 142
cradle cap on, 40
eruptions on, 87
hair loss on, 29, 87
injuries to, 134
pain in, 37, 98, *see also* headache
scalp of, 51, 87, 109
shaking of, involuntary, 98
also see dandruff
headache, 29, 51, 87, 98, 109, 132
awakening, on, 121
children, in, 14
humming in the ear, with, 76
forehead, 121
mental exertion, from, 29, 76
noise, sensitive to, 80
sick, 63, 132
small lumps on scalp, with, 142
top of head, 121, 132
yawning and stretching, 76
healing process, stages of, 3
hearing. *See* deafness; ears
heart
action, irregularities of, 19, 123
enlargement of, 19, 111
failure of, embolus, 62
palpitation of the, 31, 53, 65, 78
pericarditis, 72

trembling about the, 123
troubles, 31, 96, 97
heartburn, 110, 143
heat, 25, 100, 117
hemorrhages, 50, 51, 118
hemorrhoidal tumors, 18
hemorrhoids, 19, 52, 64, 99, 143
hernia, 14, 30, 55
herpes, 111, 117
shingles and, 66
hip, pains, 14
hip-joint disease, 41, 55, 65, 143
hives, 123
hoarseness, 29, 53, 65, 111
homesickness, 76
hopelessness, 109
hot drinks, dread of, 88
hungry feeling, after eating, 77
hydrocephalus, 37
hypoglocemia, 128
hysteria, 80

I
incontinence. *See* urinary incontinence
indigestion, 28, 88, 110. *See also* gas
infections, 14, 20, 42
inflammation, general, 50, 53, 67
injuries, 42, 54, 60
insanity, 76
insect stings, 111
intestinal worms, 37
iron phosphate. *See* Ferrum Phos
iron, deficiency of, 49

J
jaundice, 64, 110, 128, 132
jaw, 19, 25, 100
jealousy, 120
joints, 28
cracking of, 111
creaking in, 123
enlargement of, 20
lameness of, rheumatic, 53
rheumatism in, 31, 111, 123
suppuration in, 47

K
Kali Mur (potassium chloride), 62
Astrology of, Gemini, 73
burns, relieves affects of, 63
Deficiency Symptoms, 66
Disease Conditions, 66
Facial Signs of Deficiency, 66
Materia Medica, 63
Modalities, 66
Organ and Tissue Affinities, 66
Summary, 66
swellings in general, controlled, 72

Therapeutic Index, 67
Kali Phos (potassium phosphate), 74
　Astrology of, Aries, 85
　brain cells, builder of, 74
　Deficiency Symptoms, 79
　Disease Conditions, 79
　exhaustion, great, 79
　Materia Medica, 75
　Mental Disorders, all, 75
　Modalities, 79
　nervous disorders, all kinds, 74
　Organ and Tissue Affinities, 79
　Summary, 79
　Therapeutic Index, 80
Kali Sulph (potassium phosphate), 86
　Astrology of, Virgo, 90
　Deficiency Symptoms, 89
　Disease Conditions, 89
　Facial Signs of Deficiencies, 89
　hair and scalp, found in, 86
　Materia Medica, 87
　Modalities, 89
　oil, distributor of, 86
　Organ and Tissue Affinities, 89
　oxygen, in skin cells, 87
　Summary, 89
　Therapeutic Index, 90
keloids, 144
kidney(s), 65, 128
　disease, 37
　infections, 143
　stones, 133
knees, 31, 118, 111

L

labia, abscess, 143
labor pains. *See under* pregnancy
lameness, rheumatic, 37, 53
laugh lines. *See under* wrinkles
laughing, fits of, 76
legs, 31, 65, 111, 123
leucorrhea (vaginal discharge), 30, 123
　scalding and acrid, 77, 118, 123
　watery, 118
　white milky discharge, 65
　yellow, 41, 88, 123
leukemia, 31
light, sensitivity to, 6, 14, 29, 98
limbs, 31, 100
　involuntary movements of, 96, 144
　pains in, 87
　paralysis of, 78
　ulcerations of, 47
lines. *See* wrinkles
lips
　blue, 4, 20
　cancer, 88
　chapped, 20, 67

cracked, 4, 6, 19, 20, 55
　lower, peels, 88
　paleness, 55
　small, 4, 6, 32
　sore, 123
　twitching, 99
liver, 41, 130, 133, 143
liver spots, 4, 42
lockjaw, 99, 100
lumbago, 37
lungs. *See also* respiratory tract
　abscess of, with abundant sputa, 143
　edema of, 78, 110, 117
　hemorrhages of, bright red, 53
　inflammation of, 72, 90
　pains in, rheumatic, 31
　pleurisy of, 50, 65
　pneumonia of, 50, 65, 88, 111, 143
　rattling phlegm in, 90
lupus, 29, 37, 66, 142
lying down, condition better by, 54

M

Mag Phos (magnesia phosphate), 96
　Astrology of, Leo, 106
　cramping, top remedy, 100
　Deficiency Symptoms, 100
　Disease Conditions, 100
　Facial Signs of Deficiency, 101
　Materia Medica, 97
　Modalities, 100
　neuralgic pains, any tissue, 100
　Organ and Tissue Affinities, 100
　spasmodic diseases, all, 97
　Summary, 100
　Therapeutic Index, 101
magnesia phosphate. *See* Mag Phos
maniacal moods, 51
mastitis, 143. *See also* breasts
masturbation, 29
measles, 60, 66
melancholy, 109
memory, poor, 29
meningitis, 63, 133
menses/menstrual/menstruation
　amenorrhea (lack of menses), 77
　back pain with, 30
　colic (gas) with, 77, 99, 101
　delayed in young girls, 110
　diarrhea, with 133
　discharge during,
　　dark-clotted, 65
　　profuse, 60, 77, 133
　　red, bright, 30, 53
　　thin watery, 110
　dysmenorrhea (painful) 53, 99
　face flushed with, 31
　feet sweating with, fetid, 143

frequent, 65
　hysteria, with, 77
　irregular, 77, 123
　lateness of, 88, 110
　onset of, 79
　pains with, 30, 99
　suppressed, 65
　symptoms worse during, 66
mental disorders, 75, 98
mental exertion, worse by, 79, 128
milk (mother's), poor, 31
milk moustache, 67
mind, 29
morning sickness, 53, 65, 72, 122, 133
motion, worse by, 54
mouth,
　glands, suppuration of, 142
　slime, full of, 133
　tastes in, 29, 110, 122, 133
　twitching of, 99
　white about the, 122
mucus. *See* discharges
mumps, 64, 111, 118
muscles, 14, 65

N

nails 141, 143
　hangnails, 20, 53, 78
　problems with, 6, 149
　white flecks in, 6, 32
nasal discharge. *See under* nose
Nat Mur (sodium chloride), 107
　Astrology of, Aquarius, 118
　Deficiency Symptoms, 117
　Disease Conditions, 117
　Facial Signs of Deficiency, 112
　Materia Medica, 107
　Modalities, 117
　Organ and Tissue Affinities, 117
　skin, all diseases, watery exudation,
　　111
　Summary, 117
　Therapeutic Index, 117
　water, bodily distribution of, 107
Nat Phos (natrum phosphate), 120
　acid risings, 122
　acid, balance in the body, 120
　Astrology of, Libra, 128
　candida, 128
　Deficiency Symptoms, 128
　Disease Conditions, 128
　Facial Signs of Deficiency, 123
　Materia Medica, 121
　Modalities, 128
　Organ and Tissue Affinities, 128
　Summary, 128
　Therapeutic Index, 128
　worms, all kinds, 122

Nat Sulph (natrum sulphate), 130
   Astrology of, Taurus, 135
   blood, overcharged with water, 130
   Deficiency Symptoms, 134
   Disease Conditions, 134
   Facial Signs of Deficiency, 135
   liver and pancreas, 130
   Materia Medica, 131
   Modalities, 134
   Organ and Tissue Affinities, 134
   Summary, 134
   Therapeutic Index, 135
   water, regulates, 130
natrum chloride, See Nat Mur
natrum phosphate, See Nat Phos
natrum sulphate, See Nat Sulph
nausea, sour risings, 122
neck, 51, 106, 111
nerve pain, See neuralgia
nerves, 12, 14, 97
nervous system, exhausted, 75
nettle rash, 111
neuralgia (nerve pain) 31, 78, 97, 100,
   143
night sweats, 31, 143
night, symptoms worse at, 32
nodules, 31
noise, sensitivity to, 144
nose
   "alcohol nose," 135
   bell-shaped, 6
   bleeding, 14, 51, 76, 80, 109
   bluish-red coloring, 135
   congestion in the, 18, 28, 29, 88, 132
   crusts in, 109
   discharges of,
      clear, 29, 109
      foul-smelling, 18, 25
      greenish, 88
      watery, 107
      white, 64, 67
      yellow, 40, 88, 122, 142
      yellow-greenish, 67
   dryness in, 109, 132
   itching of, 122, 142
   loss of smell in, 98
   nostrils of, 29, 142
   paleness of, 55
   picking at the, 122
   polyps in, 14, 29
   pores of, black, 123
   post nasal drip of, 29
   red, dyspepsia, 128
   shiny, 4
   tip of, 29, 142
nursing, 1, 31
nutrition, poor, 32

O
Organs Affected By Cell Salt
   Deficiencies, 13
osteoporosis, 14, 32
ovaries, neuralgia of, 99

P
pain, 12, 14, 31, 78, 97. See also the
   specific body part
paleness, whole face, 4
palpitation. See heart
panic attacks, 79
pancreatic juice, 132
paralysis, 14, 74, 78
pericarditis, 72
periods, painful. See menses, dysmenorrhea
periosteum, infections of, 20
peritonitis, 60
perspiration, 32, 88, 109, 123, 143
pessimism, 74
pigmentation, 4, 6, 90
pimples. 29, 31, 40, 41, 123. See also
   acne
pleurisy, 50, 65
pneumonia, 50, 65, 88, 111, 143
pores 6, 86, 112, 123
post nasal drip, 29, 109
post traumatic stress syndrome, 76
potassium chloride, See Kali Mur
potassium phosphate, See Kali Phos
potassium sulphate, See Kali Sulph
potencies, 3
pregnancy, 1, 31
   after-pains of, 18, 19, 53
   labor pains of, 77, 99
   miscarriage during, threatening, 77
   morning sickness in, 53
pregnancy mask, face, 6, 90
penus (preputial) swelling, 133
prolapsus, any organ, 55
prostate, inflammation of, 52
puberty, pimples on face, 40
puerperal fever, 77
pulse, 53, 78, 88
purification, alchemical processes of, 7
purple shading, 4
pus, 14, 20, 144. See also suppuration
pustules, on face and neck, 144

Q
quinine, excessive use of, 112

R
rash, "rose rash," 123
rectum, prolapsed, 77
red(ness), 54
   after alcohol consumption, 6, 101

after eating 128
chronic, 4, 6, 101
embarrassment, due to, 101
face, on, 4
hairline border, on, 4, 112
"magnesium red," 101
respiratory tract, 53, 65, 77, 88
retinitis, 51, 63
rheumatic fever, 72, 90
rheumatism 37, 65, 72, 78, 134
rickets, See bone diseases
rubbing, condition better by, 25, 66

S
sacrum, burning pains in, 20
sagging, abdominal, 18
saliva, excessive, 109
salt(y)
   craving for, 110
   mucus, 109
   water, for bathing, 112
scabs, 41, 47
scales. See under skin
scalp, 109, 111, 142, see also head
scarlet fever, 47, 66, 72
scars/scarring, 14, 24, 144
sciatica, 78, 100
scoliosis, 25, 31
scrotum, 30, 143
scurvy, 66
seminal emissions, 123
sexual desire, 30, 77, 79
shins, 31
shine, 4
   gelatinous, 4, 112
   glassy, 4, 149
   greasy, 4, 6
   polished, 4, 149
   reflective, 4, 20
shingles, 111
shivering, 32
shocks, pains of, 31
shoulder blade pain, 64
shyness, 76
sighing, 31, 76
sight, loss of , 29, 51
silica. See Silicea
Silicea (silica), 141
   Astrology of, Sagittarius, 149
   Deficiency Symptoms, 144
   Disease Conditions, 144
   Facial Signs of Deficiency, 144
   Materia Medica, 142
   Modalities, 144
   Organ and Tissue Affinities, 144
   stinky feet and, 144
   Summary, 144
   suppuration and, process of, 141

surgeon of the Human Organism, 141
    sweaty hands and, 144
    Therapeutic Index, 149
    wrinkles and, 144
sinus problems, 66
sit(ting) still, inability to, 111
Skin Appearance Indicating
    Deficiencies, 4
Skin Color, all Salts, 4
skin
    appearance,
        ash-gray, 79
        fatty, 123
        gelatinous, 112
        greasy, 6
        milky, 4, 6, 67
        reflective, 20
        rosy, 135
        spongy, 112
        waxy, 6, 32
        yogurt, 32
    blackheads, 123
    blisters, watery, 111

    cancer, 37. See also face cancer
    cells, elastic fiber of, 18
    chafed, 31
    chapping, 14
    coloring, see individual colors
    combination, 6
    cracking, 14, 25
    dandruff, 14
    deposits, 6
    destruction of the, 87
    discharges,
        clear and thick, 31
        irritating, 78
        watery contents, 111
        white matter, 66
        yellow, 134, 143
        watery exudation, 111
    dry, 6, 111, 112
    eruptions, primary remedy, 72
    eyebrows, under, 4
    fragile, 14
    hard and horny, 20
    heals slowly, 143
    infections, inflammatory stage, 53
    itchy, 31, 78
    liver spots, 4, 42
    nerve spots, 6
    pigmentation, brownish-yellow, 4
    rash, 111
    scales,
        greasy, 78
        moist yellowish, 134
        powdery, 63
        white, 6, 72

sweaty, 6
    tissue, supports the, 39
    vaccinations, diseases from, 66
sleep, 14, 32, 112, 122
sleeplessness, 54, 76, 79, 144
sleepwalking, 76, 79
small pox, 54, 72, 111
smell, loss of, 98, 109
sneezing, 109
solitude, desire for, after grief, 29
spasmodic condition, 96, 97
spasms, in any tissue, 100
speaking, with teeth closed, 99
speech, stammering/spasmodic, 99
spider veins, red, 4
spina bifida, 32
spinal cord, wasting of, 66
spinal meningitis, 133
spine, curvature of the, 31
spitting, 109
splinters, 144
sprains, 53
squinting, 29, 98, 122
stings, insect, 111
stomach
    digestive conditions in, 30, 64, 67, 77,
        97, 122
    inflammation of the, 55
    pain (or spasm) in, 30, 52, 97, 99.
        See also stomachache
    ulceration in, 122
stomachache, 64, 77, 118
stool
    green and slimy, 30
    bilious, 133
    dry, 110
    food undigested in, 52
    hot, "noisy," 30
    light-colored, 64
    offensive-smelling, 30
    urging, frequent, 30,122
    watery, 110
    yellow, pale, 64
strains, 53
stretching and weariness, 79
stupor, 109
sty, 142
suffocation, 29
sugar cravings, 100, 128
suicide, 120, 132, 134
sun sensitivity, 14
sunstroke, 107, 109
suppuration, 39, 42, 149. See also
    chapters 5; 14
sweat, 6, 112, 117, 144
swelling (edema), 72. See also specific
    body part
    anemia, from, 37

blood, loss of, from, 54
    control of, 65
    hard, 17, 18, 25
    heart disease, from, 20
    smooth, 134
    soft, 63
syphilis, 19, 41 72, 110, 133

T
taste, 11, 122
tear duct, 109, 142
tears, 78
teeth
    cavities/decay, 14, 19, 37
    chattering of, 76
    dentition, slow, 29
    enamel of, 13, 14, 17, 19, 25
    grinding of, 122, 123
    loose, 19
    pain, see toothache
    roots of, 40
    tips translucent, 4, 6, 20, 32
    white flecks in, 6, 32
teething. See under children
temperature. See body temperature
temples, sunken, 4, 79
testicles, 19, 30, 65
tetanus, (lockjaw) 106
thirst, 110
thirstless, 88
thought, incapacity for, 29
throat, 52, 77
    dry, 51
    pain in swallowing, 29
    patches, white or gray, 64
    red, inflamed, 52
    sore, 41, 47, 122, 133
    spasms, 99
    ulcerations, 143
    uvula of, elongation of, 19
thrush, 109, 117
tinnitis, 60
Tissues Affected by Cell Salt
    Deficiencies, 13
tissues, hardening of, 17
Tongue Symptoms of Cell Salt
    Deficiencies, 15
tongue
    coating of,
        brownish mustard, 76, 85
        clear mucus, 109
        creamy moist, 122
        grayish-white, 64
        greenish gray, 133
        greenish-brown, 132
        white, 63
        yellow slimy, 88, 90
    cracked, 19

tongue (cont.)
  cyst under, 109
  "dirty" looking, 135
  dryness of, 76
  frothy at edge of, 109
  hardening of, 19, 143
  inflammation of, 64
  numb and stiff, 29
  red, 52
  slimy frothy, 112
  swelling of, 19
  tip, blisters or pimples on, 29
  whitish edge, 88
tonsils, 29, 63, 64, 122
tonsillitis, 41, 52, 73, 143
tooth decay, 29
toothache
  cheeks and, 19, 60
  cold liquids and, 52
  cool air and, 88
  feet chilling and, 143
  gums and, 64, 73, 85
  mental labor and 76
  pain, 99, 142
  saliva and, 109
  ulceration and, 143
  worse in evening/night, 29, 88
topical applications, 2
trigeminal neuralgia. *See* faceache
tumors
  fibroid, 62
  encysted, 18, 20
  hemorrhoidal, 18
typhoid, 42

U

ulcers, 20, 65, 73
urinary incontinence, 37, 52
urinating
  burning after, 52, 110
  frequent, 30, 77, 122
  painful when straining, 99
urine
  brick-dust appearance, 133
  dark yellow, 30, 52, 65
  egg-white appearance, 30
  flow, excessive, 19, 30, 110
  gravel sediment in, 30
  inability to retain, 122
  pus in, 143
  quantity of, increased, 19
  scalding, 77

white thick, 64
uterus, 19
  aching in, 30
  congestion of, 65, 73
  hemorrhages of, 18
  inflammation of, 53
  weakness of, 30
uvula. *See* throat

V

vaccinations, 66, 144
vaccine, poisoned by, 12
vagina
  discharges, *see* leucorrhea
  dryness in, 110
  itching of, 31
  soreness of, after urinating, 110
  spasm in, with dryness, 53
vaginal douches, 110
varicocele, 52
vein(s),
  strengthen, to, 50
  ulcerations, lower limbs, 20
  varicose, 14, 17, 19, 60
  walls, 13
vertigo, 29
  blood flow and, 60
  exhaustion and, 76
  giddiness and, 132
  heart pressure and, 133
  nervous causes of, 85
  nosebleed and, 51
vision, 18, 98
vitiligo, 4
vocal cords, paralysis of, 77
voice,
  loss of , 64, 65, 77
  shrill, sudden, 100
vomit(ing)
  after cold drinks, 30
  of blood, 52
  constriction of stomach and, 99
  green appearance before, 135
  persistent, 52
  undigested food and, 19, 52
  watery, 110
vulva, itching of 110

W

walking, condition better by, 89
walking in sleep. *See* sleepwalking
warmth 32, 42, 133, 144

warts, 111
waste substances, elimination of, 108
wasting diseases, 78
water
  accumulations of, 111
  bodily circulation of, 107
  elimination of excess, 131
  lack of, 107
  retention of, 20
  use of, 134
  water-logged condition, 131
weakness 32, 117
weariness, 75, 76
weeps easily, 109
wet cold, symptoms worse from, 13
white alabaster appearance, 4
white flecks in nails, *see* nails
white-gypsum appearance, 42
whitish, creamy look, 32
whooping cough, 31, 37, 77
  expectoration with, 65, 88
windpipe, 99, 110
womb, falling of the, 17
worms, 37, 73, 118, 122
wounds, 41, 42, 143
wrinkles, 4, 6, 20, 144
writer's cramp, 100

Y

yawning, 79, 100
yellow, 123, 132
yellow fever, 131
yellow to red coloring, 4
yellowish secretions, 87
yellowish-white crusts, 31

Z

zodiac,
  symbols of purification, 7, 9
  Aquarius, 118
  Aries, 85
  Cancer, 25
  Capricorn, 38
  Gemini, 73
  Leo, 106
  Libra, 128
  Pisces, 60
  Sagittarius, 149
  Scorpio, 47
  Taurus, 135
  Virgo, 90

ADDITIONAL INFORMATION

A poster-size version of the Zodiac/Cell Salt illustration, see page 9 in this text, is available through *Dave's Health & Nutrition* at three locations. Call or fax your orders to any store:

1108 E. 3300 S., Salt Lake City, Utah, (801) 483-9024, Fax (801) 483-9052

7777 S. State Street, Midvale, Utah, (801) 255-3809, Fax (801) 566-2725

1817 W. 9000 S, West Jordan, Utah, (801) 446-0499, Fax (801) 446-0582

About the Author

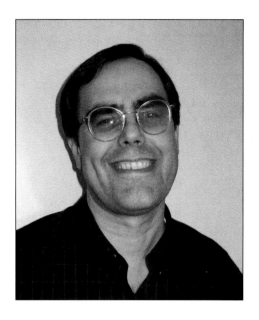

David R. Card is a certified nutritionist with a bachelor's degree in psychology from the University of Utah. He has been involved in the health and nutrition industry since 1980. Over the last twenty-five years he has graduated as a certified homeopath from the Hahnemann Academy of North America, under the direction of Dr. Robin Murphy, N.D., and has completed his first degree in herbology from the School of Natural Healing.

Dave is a native of Alberta, Canada, growing up in a family with all boys. He now lives in Salt Lake City, Utah, and is surrounded by women: his beautiful wife Teresa and their two daughters.

Dave is currently working on other books, including *Seven Symbols of Healing and Testing*. He has worked with thousands of clients using kinesiology and his expertise to help better their lives. He continues to research and study, sharing new information with students in his many classes and seminars on natural healing and homeopathy. Dave teaches both in his stores and in local colleges and schools. He is available for classes and seminars by calling (801) 483-9024.